THE EASY CANNABIS COOKBOOK

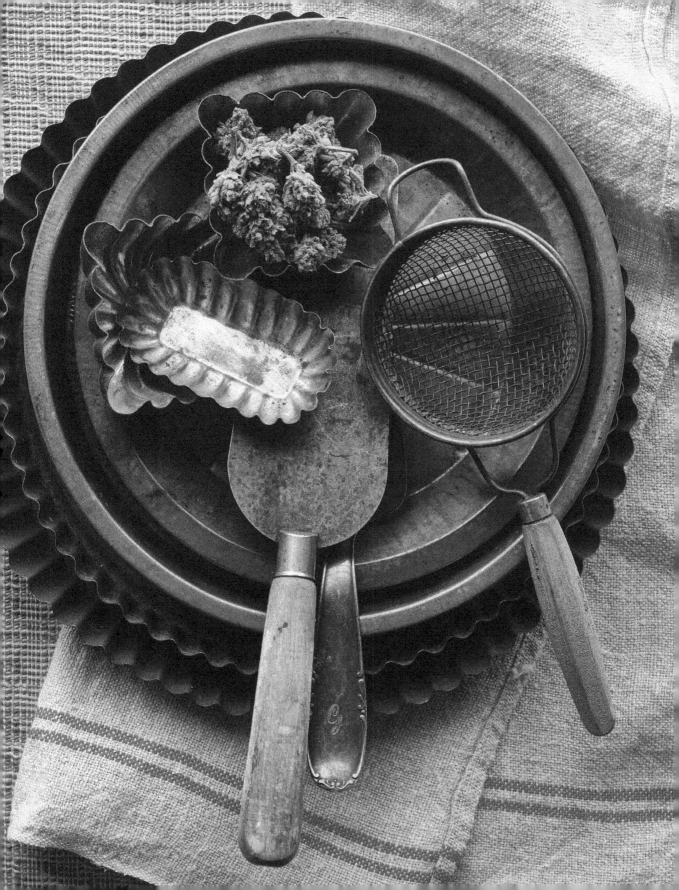

THE
EASY
CANNABIS
COOKBOOK

60+ MEDICAL MARIJUANA RECIPES
FOR SWEET AND SAVORY EDIBLES

CHERI SICARD

**ROCKRIDGE
PRESS**

FOR MY BEST FRIEND AND "BROTHER OF ANOTHER MOTHER," MITCH MANDELL, WHO HAS BRAVELY TAKEN THIS JOURNEY OUT OF THE CANNABIS CLOSET AND THROUGH THE LOOKING GLASS RIGHT ALONG WITH ME.

Rockridge Press publishes its books in a variety of electronic and print formats. Some content that appears in print may not be available in electronic books, and vice versa.

TRADEMARKS: Rockridge Press and the Rockridge Press logo are trademarks or registered trademarks of Callisto Media Inc. and/or its affiliates, in the United States and other countries, and may not be used without written permission. All other trademarks are the property of their respective owners. Rockridge Press is not associated with any product or vendor mentioned in this book.

Note: This book is intended for informational purposes only and for adults only. Neither the author, the Publisher, nor anyone else associated with this book advocates breaking the law. Marijuana laws and penalties vary substantially from country to country, state to state, and sometimes even by county and city within states where marijuana and/or medical marijuana is legal. The reader is strongly advised to read, stay up to date with, and follow the cannabis laws in their area.

Photography © Marija Vidal, cover; Lew Robertson/Stockpotimages.com, p. ii; Bettina Chavez/Stockpotimages.com, p. x; Lew Robertson/Stockpotimages.com, p. 2 & back cover; Tatevosian Yan/Shutterstock.com, p. 8; Bud_Shots/Stockpotimages.com, p. 14; DeLima/Stockpotimages.com, p. 22; Luisa Rupenian/Stockpotimages.com, p. 32; Kostrez/Shutterstock.com, p. 34; Laniak, Malgorzata/Stockfood, p. 48; Renée Comet/Stockfood, p. 64; J.R. Photography/Stocksy, p. 78; Susan Brooks-Dammann/Stocksy, p. 100; Shannon Douglas, p. 114; Cameron Zegers/Stocksy, p. 134.

ISBN: Print 978-1-93975-432-5
eBook 978-1-93975-433-2

CONTENTS

INTRODUCTION

WITH ALL THE HYSTERIA, hype, and complicated legal wrangling surrounding marijuana, it's easy to lose sight of the fact that *Cannabis sativa*, a.k.a. ganja, weed, grass, *mota*, Mary Jane, and a host of other monikers, is nothing more than a simple plant that grows wild and free in nature.

Enlightened humans have been using cannabis for medical, spiritual, and recreational purposes since before recorded history. And for almost as long, other humans have demonized and stigmatized the plant and its users in order to advance their own agendas, whether by gaining political control, furthering financial interests, or a combination of the two.

While no amount of fabricated reefer madness could kill the popularity of this incredible plant, millennia of misinformation have led people to form some pretty wild misconceptions, which in turn kept marijuana from entering the mainstream . . . until now.

With substantial help from the Internet, the truth about marijuana's healing and disease-prevention properties is finally reaching the masses, and reefer madness is being exposed for just what it is—agenda-based propaganda with little basis in fact.

As more research and credible information comes to light and more states legalize marijuana for medicinal or recreational purposes, modern consumers are becoming quite sophisticated about their cannabis use. While simple joint-passing at a party still occurs, today's cannabis consumers are just as likely to eschew smoking entirely in favor of vaporizing or eating their marijuana.

Edible cannabis makes logical sense; after all, we are talking about a plant, and, like many other green plants, marijuana is an antioxidant-rich superfood that can help prevent certain diseases and ease the symptoms of others.

The effects of edible cannabis take longer to manifest, but they last far longer than smoking or vaping and likewise can help stretch your marijuana budget. You can also expect to feel the effects of edible marijuana more profoundly—a very good thing, especially if you are dealing with conditions like chronic pain or insomnia.

Why should you bother making your own edibles, as opposed to buying them in a dispensary (if you are lucky enough to live where that is even an option)? Besides the obvious cost advantage, making your own allows you to medicate the food you like to eat with the exact dose that works best for you.

Most commercial edibles tend to be cookies, brownies, and candies, but there is nothing magical about sweets that necessitates they be the primary vehicle for the cannabis. And while there's nothing wrong with treats in moderation, medical marijuana patients and those who use "medibles" every day are going to start looking for healthier fare and a wider variety. The best way to get these is to make them yourself.

Almost any recipe can be successfully infused with cannabis . . . if you know how to do it. This book is going to teach you everything you need to know, including the most important but challenging part of cannabis cooking: proper dosing.

When I first started cooking with cannabis, I made an educated guess as to how much to use. My edibles usually came out too heavily dosed. In fact, one of my first batches of cookies caused most of my friends to sleep through an entire three-day music festival!

People's dosing needs are different, and not just a little bit different—DRASTICALLY different. Ten milligrams of THC is too much for some people, while others will need 100 milligrams or more to feel anything. When you make edibles yourself, you can customize them to deliver the exact effects you want, as your preferences may change for various times and occasions.

Cannabis cooking is not difficult once you understand a few basic principles. It takes no special tools or gadgets—chances are you already have everything you need. This book will complete the puzzle and teach you the essential information you need in order to get safe and satisfying results. You'll also find tons of quick and easy-to-make cannabis recipes, not just sweet treats but delicious, savory foods you can enjoy any time of day.

Now, let's get cooking with cannabis.

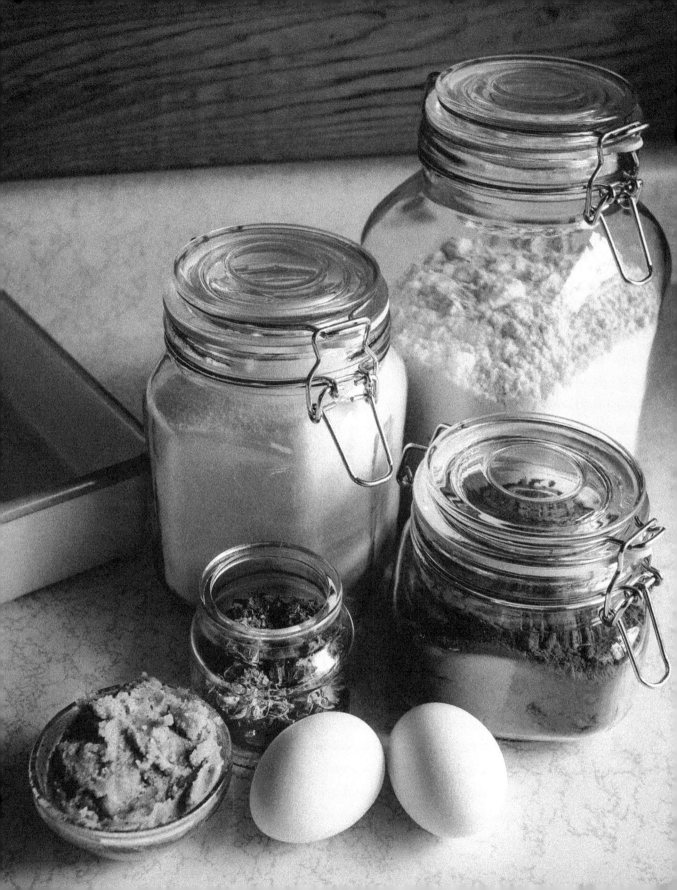

PART 1
THE CANNABIS KITCHEN

Chances are, you already have a cannabis kitchen, it just lacks cannabis.

Before you dig into the recipes in part 2, there are a few basics to cover first, and this section of the book does it in three parts:

WHAT—What cannabis and cannabis edibles are and what you can expect when making and consuming them

WHERE—Where and how to find cannabis for cooking at the best value

HOW—How to combine essential skills and knowledge to make perfect marijuana edibles every time you cook

If you are reading this book, I trust you already know the WHY: Because cannabis is a unique superfood that can dramatically improve your health and quality of life.

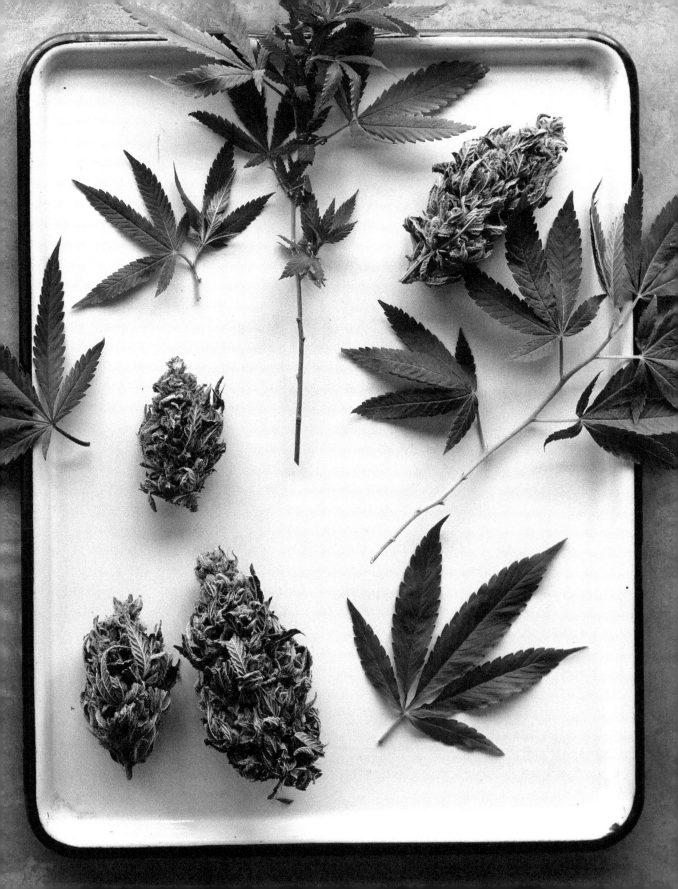

CHAPTER 1
CANNABIS HERB

Before you start cooking, let's briefly examine the incredible plant you will be working with. No other individual species of flora has been so misunderstood. Some malign it, exaggerating and even inventing all manner of fear-mongering propaganda. Others laud it as a miracle cure for anything and everything that ails humanity and the planet. Like most polarizing topics, the truth is somewhere in between those two extremes.

A BRIEF HISTORY OF CANNABIS EDIBLES

Our ancient ancestors had a far more intimate relationship with food as medicine than most of us do today. Many plants familiar to us, including basil, cinnamon, cumin, fennel, mint, oregano, thyme, and cannabis, were intertwined in both kitchen and apothecary throughout history.

Our earliest written references to cannabis appear around the fifteenth century BCE in China, where it was consumed as a tea. However, scholars agree that surviving ancient medical texts speak of cannabis use in the past tense, giving the impression that it had been a common medical staple long before written texts confirmed the fact.

By 1000 BCE, cannabis (or *bhang*) was being cultivated in India, where the Vedas, collections of Hindu religious texts, considered it one of five sacred plants. In addition to referring to the plant itself, bhang is the name of arguably the world's oldest marijuana recipe, an ancient cannabis-laced drink that remains popular in India today. During the Middle Ages, soldiers customarily consumed bhang for fortification before going off into battle.

Even though cannabis is technically illegal in India today, bhang is still sold, especially during the Hindu Holi festival when it is such an essential, traditional part of the celebration that the government has found it easier to turn a blind eye than fight it.

Around 1474, Bartolomeo Platina put the first cannabis recipe into print in what is considered the world's oldest known cookbook. Platina advised his readers on making cannabis-infused oil, not unlike what we do today (see page 38).

Moroccan ancients consumed their cannabis in the form of hashish, as referenced in the original collection of folk tales *One Thousand and One Nights* (also known as *The Arabian Nights*). An ancient Middle Eastern marijuana recipe still popular today is *mahjoun*. This uncooked jam features dates, nuts, honey, spices, and hashish rolled into bite-sized balls—and provides a healthier sweet than most of today's infused edibles.

In the 1840s, Europe's intellectual, literary, and artistic elite gathered in Paris's Club des Hachischins (Club of the Hashish-Eaters) to consume hash in their coffees and teas and via infused tinctures.

Prior to Prohibition (1920–1933), most American medicine cabinets contained cannabis, usually in the form of tinctures, but edible candies and other foods also proliferated, broadening the market. An 1862 issue of *Vanity Fair* magazine carried an ad touting the the Gunjah Wallah Company's "Hasheesh Candy" as a "medicinal agent for the cure of nervousness, weakness, [and] melancholy."

EDIBLE CANNABIS: A TIME LINE

15TH CENTURY BCE
The Chinese consume cannabis tea.

CIRCA 2000 TO 1400 BCE
The Indian Vedas consider cannabis, or bhang, one of five sacred plants.

CIRCA 1474 CE
The world's first known cookbook is released and includes a marijuana recipe.

16TH CENTURY CE
Cannabis is cultivated throughout Morocco.

Alice B. Toklas, life partner of author Gertrude Stein, ushered in the era of modern edibles while simultaneously resurrecting *mahjoun*'s popularity for modern generations when she published her recipe for Haschich Fudge in *The Alice B. Toklas Cookbook* (1954).

Toklas's recipe uses ground bud and contains no hash. It resembles neither fudge nor brownies, despite it entering the popular lexicon as "Alice B. Toklas Brownies," thanks to the 1968 Peter Sellers film *I Love You, Alice B. Toklas*. In the movie, Sellers's uptight attorney character consumes a pot brownie that forever alters his world. The movie permanently changed the public's perception of marijuana edibles, and from that point on the "pot brownie" became embedded in the mainstream consciousness as the most popular way to consume edible cannabis.

But history is always in the making, and since the experience of edible marijuana is about so much more than pot brownies, I think it's time to create new history. This book will teach you how.

THE UNSUNG SUPERFOOD

While the word "superfood" is assuredly more a marketing term than a medical one, it does refer to nutrient-dense foods, usually plant-based, that are shown to bring health benefits when consumed. By this definition, marijuana qualifies as one of the planet's most powerful superfoods, even without taking into account all the illnesses cannabis can combat and prevent.

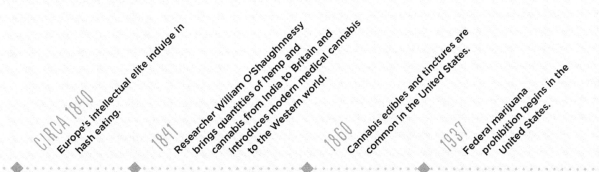

CIRCA 1840
Europe's intellectual elite indulge in hash eating.

1841
Researcher William O'Shaughnessy brings quantities of hemp and cannabis from India to Britain and introduces modern medical cannabis to the Western world.

1860
Cannabis edibles and tinctures are common in the United States.

1937
Federal marijuana prohibition begins in the United States.

SUPERFOOD MEDICINE

All mammals, including humans, are born with a natural form of cannabis, or endocannabinoids, in their systems. Endocannabinoids, along with cannabinoid receptors in the brain and body, make up what is known as the endocannabinoid system (ECS), which is essential for maintaining homeostasis throughout the body.

Some scientists theorize that because of the ravages of modern living, including poor diet, decreased exercise, and a prevalence of toxic chemicals in our air, water, and food, most people are now endocannabinoid deficient. Since the body's own natural endocannabinoids can't keep up with the demand needed to maintain optimum health, supplemental cannabinoids from marijuana can give it more ammunition to fight disease.

One of the world's foremost researchers on the subject, Dr. Robert Melamede, the former chair of the biology department at the University of Colorado Colorado Springs, says:

"Cannabis is an essential nutrient for modern man. The endocannabinoid system of vertebrates is a major regulator of inflammation and by increasing our endocannabinoid activity we can lower the damage caused by excessive inflammatory responses."

Cannabinoids and terpenoids are the chemical compounds within the marijuana plant responsible for its medicinal effects. Scientists have isolated over 110 cannabinoids in marijuana including THC, CBD, CBN, CBG, CBC, and many more.

EDIBLE CANNABIS: A TIME LINE CONTINUED

1954
The Alice B. Toklas Cookbook is published, including a recipe for Haschich Fudge.

CIRCA 1990
Mary Jane Rathbun, a.k.a. "Brownie Mary," illegally bakes and serves marijuana brownies to San Francisco AIDS patients. After being arrested three times, bringing international attention to the cannabis movement, the grandmotherly Rathbun was instrumental in making California the first state to legalize medical marijuana.

Terpenoids, or terpenes, give all plants—not just marijuana plants—their aromas. They also have powerful medicinal effects. Over 200 terpenes have been identified in cannabis and these, too, play an important role in the health-giving qualities of the plant. Terpenes interact with cannabinoids and are responsible for many of the nuances in how different marijuana strains make you feel.

THC

Tetrahydrocannabinol, or THC, gets all the hype because it is the component responsible for the high you feel after eating or inhaling marijuana. But there's far more to THC than just getting high, not that there is anything wrong with that—the mild euphoria that comes with a cannabis high is indeed a medicinal effect. THC can also help provide relief from pain, glaucoma, insomnia, nausea, PTSD, and a whole host of other ailments.

CBD

Cannabidiol, or CBD, is typically a nonpsychoactive cannabinoid, meaning most people will not feel high when taking it. CBD can be effective for treating seizures, anxiety, pain, inflammation, and more.

Rather than isolating CBD or THC, know that cannabis works best as a whole-plant medicine with all the terpenes and cannabinoids working together and enhancing each other's effects, something scientists call "the entourage effect." Nature designed it right, as many of the diseases treated by the various cannabinoids overlap.

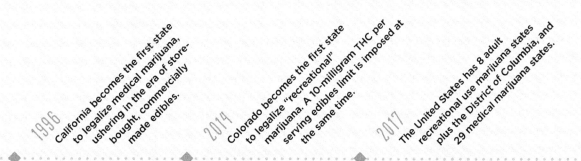

1996 California becomes the first state to legalize medical marijuana, ushering in the era of store-bought, commercially made edibles.

2014 Colorado becomes the first state to legalize "recreational" marijuana. A 10-milligram THC per serving edibles limit is imposed at the same time.

2017 The United States has 8 adult recreational use marijuana states plus the District of Columbia, and 29 medical marijuana states.

THE CANNABIS PHARMACY

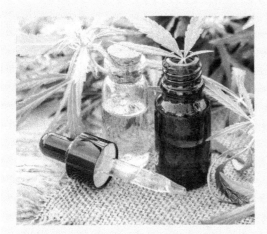

Cannabis can treat so many maladies it might be easier to list things it doesn't help, but even that would be difficult as this plant affects individuals so differently.

While politicians like to say, "We need more research," that's only partially true. Yes, we need much more research in order to better understand all the things this amazing plant can do and how to best use and administer it in clinical settings. However, we already have plenty of research proving its safety and efficacy. In fact, cannabis is one of the most studied plants on the planet. There are over 22,000 scientific studies and reviews mentioning cannabis and cannabinoids.

Here are some of the most important emerging medicinal uses of cannabis:

- Addiction treatment
- Alzheimer's disease
- Amyotrophic Lateral Sclerosis (ALS, also known as Lou Gehrig's disease)
- Cancer
- Chronic pain
- Crohn's disease
- Dementia
- Depression
- Diabetes mellitus
- Epilepsy
- Fibromyalgia
- Gastrointestinal disorders
- Hepatitis C
- HIV
- Huntington's disease
- Hypertension
- Irritable Bowel Syndrome (IBS)
- Incontinence
- Methicillin-Resistant Staphylococcus Aureus (MRSA)
- Multiple sclerosis (MS)
- Osteoporosis
- Parkinson's disease
- Post-Traumatic Stress Disorder (PTSD)
- Pruritus
- Rheumatoid arthritis
- Sleep apnea
- Tourette's syndrome

SUPERFOOD NUTRITION

While science has yet to delve into marijuana's nutritional profile, it has done so with its nonpsychoactive cousin, hemp. Since cannabis and hemp have similar genetics and come from the same species of plant, *Cannabis sativa*, it's safe to assume that cannabis can deliver the same powerful, nutritional punch of hemp, plus a whole lot more thanks to its abundance of THC, CBD, CBN, and other cannabinoids. If hemp is considered a superfood, then marijuana should be considered a super-duper food.

When it comes to edible seeds, you will want to opt for hemp simply because marijuana seeds would be cost prohibitive to chow down on, but marijuana leaves and flowers are also nutritional powerhouses, if you have a way to get them.

Let's consider some of the ways hemp and marijuana nutritionally qualify as superfoods:

Omega Fatty Acids Cannabis and hemp seeds contain omega-3 and omega-6 fatty acids that promote neurological health, ease pain, manage skin conditions, and ease symptoms of diabetic neuropathy, ADD, and ADHD.

Protein Hemp seeds pack 20 amino acids into their tiny packages, including the nine essential amino acids. A tablespoon of seeds contains 5½ grams of protein.

Vitamins and Minerals Cannabis seeds, leaves, and flowers are filled with vitamins and minerals, including beta-carotene, phosphorous, potassium, calcium, iron, zinc, and vitamins B_1, B_3, and B_6, C, and E.

Raw Mega Nutrition One of the latest trends in therapeutic healing is eating or juicing the leaves and flowers of raw cannabis plants. Dr. William Courtney, the California physician leading this charge, believes the raw form is far superior, going so far as to call cannabis the "most important vegetable on the planet."

According to Courtney, raw plant therapy can boost immune system function, provide anti-inflammatory benefits, improve bone metabolism and neural function, and even prohibit cancer growth.

The key is in the amount of cannabinoids one is able to ingest. For instance, instead of taking in 10 milligrams or so of THC like most smokers, juicing the raw leaves and flowers allows the patient to ingest up to 600 milligrams of nonpsychoactive THC-acid. Besides the fact that raw plants won't get you high, this megadose of cannabinoids and terpenoids constitutes the principal difference between what most people think of as "medical marijuana" and the new trend of "alternative dietary cannabis."

Unless you grow your own marijuana, you will never see leaves, and getting a supply of fresh organic cannabis to juice is nearly impossible. However, it will be interesting to see where the research on this new trend takes us.

PRACTICAL TIPS ON BUYING, STORING, AND PREPPING CANNABIS

Bringing marijuana home from your favorite purveyor is not like acquiring other produce as it will arrive in your hands already trimmed, dried, and ready for smoking or vaping. But there are a few things to know and do before cooking.

BUYING

Outside of growing your own marijuana, you will rarely encounter trimmings, and you will never encounter stems or fan leaves. Even if you can get them, skip the stalks, stems, and large fan leaves as the proliferation of trichomes, the small resinous glands on the surface of the plant that contain the cannabinoids and terpenes, is too small for the level of potency they add to infused ingredients.

Now that you know what not to cook with, let's explore ideal cannabis cooking materials.

- **Trimmings** include tiny, trichome-covered "sugar leaves" that surround the flower, and small "popcorn buds" that grow near the bottom of the plant. You will rarely find trimmings for sale, but if you know anyone who grows, you might be able to get a good deal on them for cooking. It never hurts to ask.
- **Shake** is an economical cooking (or smoking) product comprised of small pieces that break off large buds and filter to the bottom of a large bag of marijuana. Shake is tasty and made from the same plants, but costs a fraction of the price of flowers. Not all vendors sell shake, but many do and others can get it if they have a customer who wants it, so always ask.
- **Marijuana buds or flowers** will probably be your only option, if you don't grow your own. Don't worry, it's still more economical than buying premade edibles. There is no need to buy the most expensive top-shelf marijuana for cooking. Just ask your seller for a reasonably priced potent strain.
- **Marijuana concentrates** like kief (the resinous trichomes with little to no plant material), hash (kief that has been heated and pressed), or hash oils (concentrated oils extracted using a solvent, usually CO_2 or butane) also make terrific cooking materials, although the latter will probably not be cost effective. Decarboxylated concentrates can be stirred directly into recipes or infused into butter, oil, or other ingredients.

STORING

Properly storing marijuana will help preserve its terpenes; however, there is no such thing as a marijuana expiration date. As long as it shows no signs of mold or decay, you can cook with cannabis years after harvest and still achieve great results.

Here are some essential storage tips:

- Avoid plastic and store in an airtight glass container in a cool, dark place.
- Leave buds intact, waiting until you are ready to use them before crumbling or grinding.
- Avoid light damage by storing in a dark glass jar or storing clear jars in cool, dark cabinets.
- Marijuana's ideal humidity is 65 percent. Anything significantly lower than 50 percent can result in premature dryness, although that poses no problems for cooking. However, high humidity can result in moisture buildup and mold growth, so it is a good idea to open jars every few days if you live in a humid area. If your grower has properly cured their harvest, this won't be an issue.

PREPPING

Marijuana does not require much preparation, but there are a couple of necessary steps before you start cooking.

THE GRIND

In most every instruction you find, except mine, you'll be advised to finely grind your cooking cannabis, often using a food processor or coffee grinder. In fact, a popular commercial infused butter maker has this capability built into it with no way to bypass the function.

Don't finely grind your weed.

The resinous cannabinoid and terpenoid-filled trichomes you are extracting are *on* the plant, not *in* it. Despite asking countless experts, I have never gotten a satisfactory answer as to why so many people finely grind their marijuana besides, "That's the way we've always done it."

The only thing fine grinding accomplishes is to deposit more plant material into your cannabis infusion, which likewise means the finished edibles will have a more pronounced cannabis flavor, something most people don't like.

My recommendation is to use your fingers or a handheld grinder to break up the plant material in much the same way you would if you planned to roll it into a joint. There is no need to pulverize it into a fine powder.

DECARBOXYLATION

You might be surprised to learn that raw marijuana plants contain no THC or CBD, but instead contain the acidic form of these cannabinoids, THCa and CBDa. Both have medicinal qualities unto themselves, but most people are looking for the effects that come from the nonacidic THC and CBD. For the purposes of this book, I will assume you are, too.

It takes the process of heating, or decarboxylation, to release the carbon dioxide that causes the chemical reaction that converts THCa and CBDa into THC and CBD.

Some people get elaborate with decarboxylation and use a boil-in-bag or sous vide method. Some seal the cannabis in oven bags and bake it. There is even a special home decarbing machine on the market that promises to convert 100 percent of the THCa into THC.

It need not be so complicated. Simply place the crumbled plant material into an ovenproof dish or ramekin, cover, and bake at 250°F for about 20 minutes. Take it out of the oven and your cannabis is now decarbed and ready to use.

IS DECARBOXYLATION ALWAYS NECESSARY?

You might wonder if you need to take the extra step of decarboxylating cannabis if you are going to turn it into an infusion that you will be cooking with later. You don't have to, but you may want to.

While cannabis will partially decarboxylate during cooking, lab tests show that even when making a long-cooking infusion, you can extract a bit more potency by taking the time to decarboxylate first. The difference might not be dramatic, but if your goal is to extract the maximum amount of THC possible from your marijuana, take the time to decarboxylate. If you plan on adding marijuana flowers, or a concentrate like kief, hash, or hash oil, directly into your foods without making an infusion, you will always want to take the time to decarboxylate first.

The reliability and stability of your oven temperature can affect how much of the THCa is converted to psychoactive THC, but if you decarb and then infuse, you should be getting most, if not all, of it. Besides, any THCa left still imparts important medicinal benefits.

Those who want to make sure they convert 100 percent of the THC can invest in the NOVA, a small gadget that maintains proper time and temp to do just that. But know that a special device is not essential to decarb your cannabis and successfully make edibles.

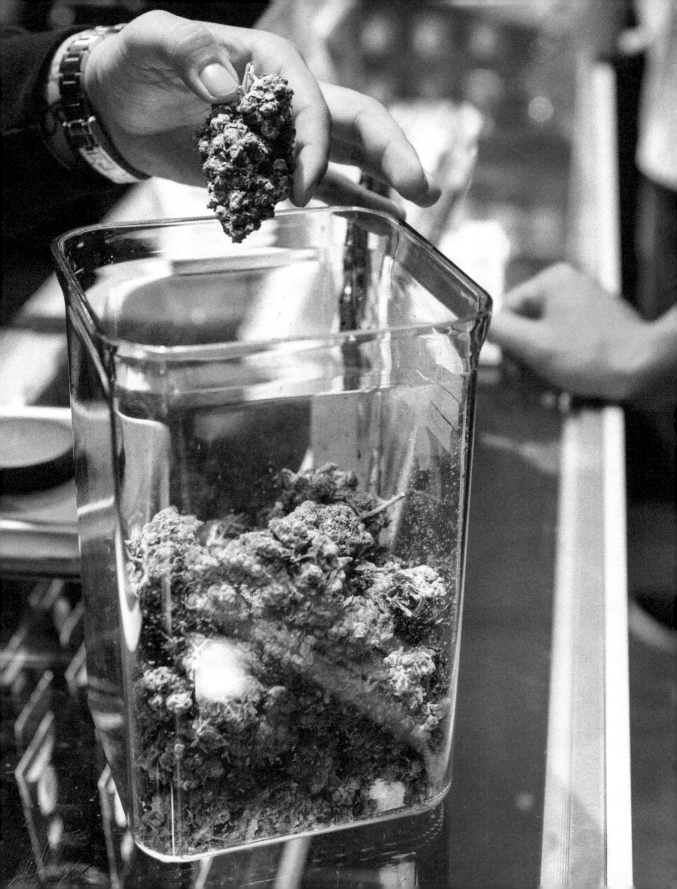

CHAPTER 2
CANNABIS DISPENSARIES

Where you live will have a major impact on how and where you procure cannabis. If you live in a state where marijuana is legal or medicinally legal, you may have the luxury of shopping at well-stocked modern dispensaries. But even within legal states there is no single dispensary experience because, at this point in our history, cannabis laws and regulations are a hodgepodge of state and local ordinances, some that contradict each other.

Some places let you examine and smell the wares before you buy, others require everything to be prepackaged and stay that way. Some areas limit dosages and potencies while others impose no restrictions. Some areas require dispensaries to grow their own cannabis while others expressly forbid it. Labeling, testing, and allowable pesticide levels also vary, not to mention the amount you'll be taxed.

Until marijuana becomes federally legal, and likely even long after, dealing with these kinds of inconsistencies is just something consumers need to do in order to legally obtain cannabis.

But let's take a look at the optimal cannabis dispensary experience.

If you have never visited a big dispensary before, it can be intimidating, but also fun. The dazzling array of flowers, concentrates, edibles, and topicals can make you feel like a kid in a candy store.

Don't be afraid to ask questions. A good dispensary will have a knowledgeable staff who are willing to take time to explain the merchandise and help you find what you need. If your dispensary doesn't provide that, shop around until you find one that does.

GROWERS

Arguably the most important, yet least appreciated, person in the cannabis food chain, the grower controls the raw product, how potent it is, what kind of yield it offers, the presence or lack of pesticides and other contaminants, and more. As with any other consumable commodity, it's a good idea to know as much as possible about how your cannabis was grown.

WHO?

If you live in an area that requires dispensaries to grow their own cannabis, it will be easy to get information about how it was grown. If you don't, you may or may not have access to accurate information.

Most dispensaries obtain their cannabis from multiple growers. Sources can and do change frequently. Just because last month's harvest was top shelf does not mean next month's will be. Likewise dispensary buyers are constantly on the lookout for the best products at the most competitive prices. These might come from a company maintaining a warehouse-sized industrial grow, or it might come from a single entrepreneurial individual or family farm.

As this burgeoning industry evolves and comes out of the shadows, it will become more transparent about who grows the marijuana. You can already see it happening in thriving cannabis markets such as California and Colorado, where things are so competitive that farms and growers are investing in serious branding campaigns. We are even starting to see small farmers banding together in cooperatives, much like the wine industry does with grape-growing cooperatives.

WHAT?

Choosing cannabis has a lot in common with wine tasting, so you have to try a lot of different kinds in order to discover what you like best. (Oh, darn.)

Consumer demand can fuel product production, such as the trends toward organically grown marijuana and CBD-rich strains. The number of strains lining dispensary shelves boggles the mind. Some are long-standing favorites like Blue Dream, Cookies and Cream, and OG Kush, others have names made up on the spot for marketing purposes by the dispensary owner.

Until there is standardization in the industry, strains present a tricky road for consumers to navigate. California testing lab The Werc Shop tested thousands of samples from that state and found the results varied widely. What one purveyor called "OG Kush" often had a completely different terpene and cannabinoid profile from what another shop claimed was the same variety.

With so many variables involved, your best option is to find a good dispensary and stick with it. As The Werc Shop found, what it says on the bottle may or may not be accurate, but if you find a strain you like, chances are the same dispensary will get it from the same grower again. If you source the same strain elsewhere, it might be different.

Choosing marijuana need not be so complicated, however, unless you choose to study strains. Know that you can successfully cook with any type or strain of cannabis and get great results.

WHERE?

The majority of dispensary marijuana is grown indoors, as this method allows gardeners to consistently turn out crop after crop year-round. Indoor cultivation also gives the grower complete control over the plant's environment, including light, food, and water.

Outdoor growers get a single chance to get their crop right. If the garden falls prey to pests, foul weather, or thieves, it's all over until the next year. Perhaps that's why premium, outdoor sun-grown cannabis—especially from famous growing regions in California, like Humboldt and Mendocino, that treat it as an art—have devoted followings that anxiously await each annual harvest.

Sadly, at this time in such a young industry, there are no standard practices. Regulations are left to the same patchwork of local and state laws that govern all cannabis commerce. While some states and regions within states tightly regulate how cannabis is produced, others leave far more to chance—further reason to seek out quality purveyors you can trust and stick with them.

SHOULD YOU GROW YOUR OWN?

There's no better way to know exactly what is, and isn't, in your cannabis than to grow it yourself. If you enjoy gardening, cannabis cultivation could be a fun and satisfying hobby. Outdoor growing is not difficult and you can even get good results in a large container on a discreet, sunny apartment balcony. Indoor growing takes more time and tinkering, but if you enjoy this sort of activity you will be well rewarded for your efforts.

However, cannabis cultivation is not for everyone. Before you go any further, ask yourself these questions:

Do you have the space? Outdoors, you will need a childproof, sunny space away from nosy eyes. Indoors, you'll require a special light-tight room, or space to put a portable grow tent big enough to hold your plants.

Do you have the time? Besides the initial time you'll spend studying your grow method of choice, each indoor crop will take between 8 to 14 weeks, depending on the strain. Outdoors, plan on working from May through October, in addition to preparing soil and starting seedlings or clones in advance.

Do you have the money? You can grow some respectable outdoor marijuana with an investment of $100 or less depending on what you already have on hand. Plan to spend between $500 to $3,000 (plus electricity costs) for your small indoor grow, depending on how much equipment and buildout you need and whether you plan on growing in soil or hydroponically (in water).

Do you have the chutzpah? No matter what the local laws in your area, as long as it is federally illegal, growing marijuana always carries some risk.

SAVVY BUYER TIPS

Can buying marijuana be as simple as walking into a store and walking out with weed, or calling a delivery service and having it arrive at your door an hour later? Yes, it can, if you live in the right area and have taken the proper preliminary steps.

WHAT TO DO (BEFORE YOU GO)

Pre-trip planning before heading to a dispensary depends on where you live. If you are in one of the recreationally legal states, you can simply walk in the door, prove you are of legal age, and walk out with marijuana.

If you are in a medicinally legal state, you will need to obtain a doctor's recommendation in order to legally purchase and possess cannabis. Notice the doctor's recommendation is *not* called a "prescription" as federal law prohibits doctors from prescribing Schedule I substances.

The legal landscapes of medical marijuana states are as varied as their geographical terrains. The most restrictive severely limit the illnesses that qualify for a recommendation, while in others almost any health complaint, major or minor, will qualify. While prohibitionists like to scoff at this, cannabis can help with more than just catastrophic health conditions, providing all-natural relief for everything from minor aches and pains to menstrual cramps, occasional insomnia, and much more.

Make sure you have your medical marijuana credentials in order and bring them with you to the dispensary along with a photo ID. Unless you know otherwise, bring cash, too. Because of federal prohibition, most banks refuse to service the cannabis industry even in legal states, so most transactions are done in cash.

WHAT TO EXPECT

Some medical states have no dispensaries whatsoever, while in others consumers can find marijuana megamarts stocked with endless varieties of flowers, concentrates, edibles, and topicals. Some even have ancillary merchandise like books, smoking and vaping supplies, and accessories.

It's not uncommon for dispensaries to offer new patient bonuses, such as an edible or joint, or frequent buyer rewards much like a coffee shop. Some also arrange demo days with growers and manufacturers so patients can check out new products and get their questions answered, usually along with a substantial discount on the product being featured.

Regardless of which state you live in, the best dispensaries:

* Are clean and well lit.
* Have on-site security (because of zoning laws, dispensaries are often relegated to less-than-ideal areas of town).

- Have knowledgeable staff members, familiar with the merchandise, who can make recommendations based on your needs.
- Stock a variety of quality merchandise at a fair price.
- Offer lab-tested cannabis and professionally produced edibles and topicals.

Award a dispensary extra points if they offer educational or community outreach programs.

DISPENSARY BUYER TIPS

As with any specialty industry, there are things you can do to have the best buying experience:

- The more you buy, the cheaper it gets. The price per gram will be far less if you buy an ounce than if you buy an eighth. Some dispensaries offer greater discounts on quarter pounds. Go in with a friend and save big bucks.
- If your dispensary offers "patient appreciation days," there will be bargains and most likely free samples, too.
- If you find a good dispensary, be loyal to it and get to know the staff. Once they know what you like, they'll make recommendations of new products and good deals, and often let you sample them.
- Being a regular can have other rewards. For instance, PureLife Alternative Wellness in Chatsworth, California, sells shake for a mere $30 an ounce, but only to regular customers.

Signs you are in a less-than-ideal dispensary:

- The store is dirty or unkempt.
- The staff is uninterested in helping you with choices.
- The merchandise is old or not professionally packaged or produced.
- There is no menu or price list.
- If you feel unsafe for any reason, based on the staff, other customers, the location, whatever—leave.

When it comes to asking questions at dispensaries, it is only as valuable as the level of knowledge of the person answering. If your dispensary has a passionate, well-trained staff, you can learn a lot. If they don't, you might get bad information and leave more confused than when you arrived.

Inquire as to how the cannabis you are interested in was grown. Does the farmer use organic practices? Is it grown indoors or outdoors? What does the budtender—the person who works behind the dispensary's counter—know about its potency and effects?

Lab testing, too, is only as good as the lab that did the testing and the technician who performed the test. This is another area of the industry that needs standardization as there are many variables, and so far it has been rife with scandal, like results skewing in favor of high-paying clients, or producers who cut corners by not testing each new crop. Lab testing can tell you a lot, as long as it is an accurate test.

LEGALIZING MARIJUANA

The federal government continues to classify cannabis as a Schedule I drug, the definition of which states it "has no accepted medical value and has a high potential for abuse," both demonstrably false claims.

As of this writing, Alaska, California, Colorado, Maine, Massachusetts, Oregon, Washington, and the District of Columbia have legalized cannabis for adult recreational use. Twenty-nine states have legalized some form of medical marijuana. Both categories are expected to increase their roster with each new election cycle.

Marijuana laws are in constant flux, and vary dramatically from state to state and even within different regions within states. Always consult with your state, county, and local laws in order to stay as legally compliant as possible, especially before growing your own. Despite strong public support of legalization, law enforcement has been slow to catch up, so marijuana users often have to fight to protect their own rights.

Keep up with the latest in marijuana law at the National Organization for the Reform of Marijuana Law's website, where you can also keep abreast of the latest medical research: NORML.org.

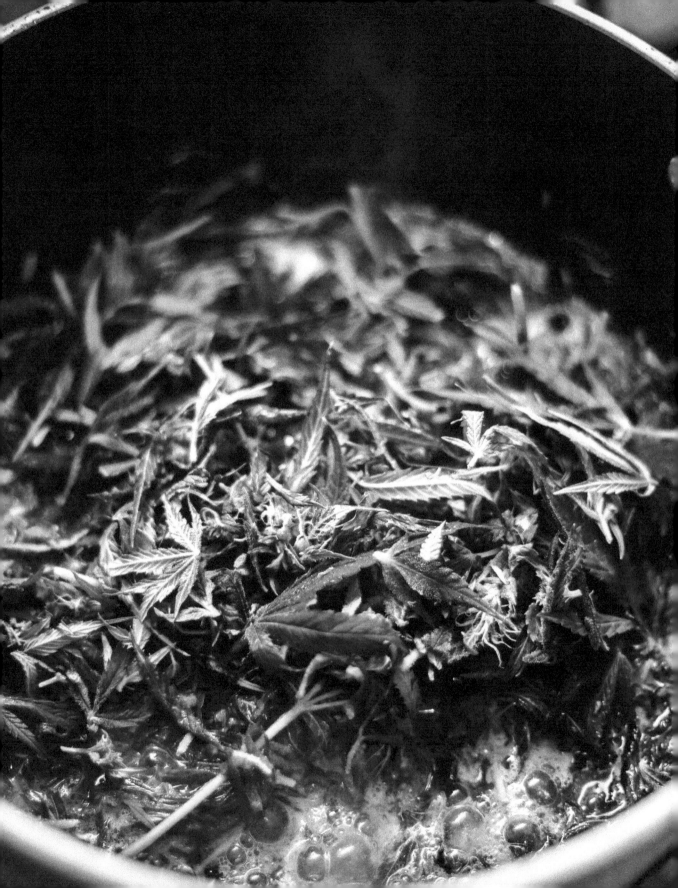

CHAPTER 3
CANNABIS STAPLES & POTENCY

Think of this chapter as the detailed instructions for the recipes in part 2 of this book. It will bring you up to speed with the basics before you actually get down to making infusions and cooking with cannabis.

CANNABIS STAPLES

Infusions form the backbone of cannabis cooking, as most marijuana recipes call for a quantity of infused cannabis butter, cooking oil, or other staple (such as honey, cream, syrups, or alcohol) which in turn are mixed with other ingredients.

In chapter 4, you'll find specific recipes and instructions for making staples using the methods below.

RECOMMENDED INFUSION-MAKING METHODS

Every cannabis cook has his or her favorite method of making infusions. It really is a matter of personal preference, what material you are infusing, and the amount you are making. Yes, if you are *very careful* you can infuse over direct heat on the stove top, but

I usually tell people to avoid this as it is far too easy to render the whole thing useless by burning or overheating. Instead, try one of these easier infusion methods:

SLOW COOKER

My personal favorite infusing tool is a slow cooker.

PROS	CONS
• Requires little to no monitoring. Simply stir in cannabis along with the oil or butter and walk away for hours.	• Requires buying a separate gadget if you don't already have one, albeit an inexpensive one that will last for many years.
• Maintains a steady low temperature.	
• Pretty much foolproof.	

STOVE-TOP INDIRECT HEAT VIA DOUBLE BOILER

In the absence of a slow cooker, the indirect heat on the stove top is your next best option.

A **double boiler** suspends a pot containing the plant material and infusion medium over another pot of simmering water. If you don't have a double boiler, you can improvise one by simmering water in a stockpot and suspending a covered saucepan over it.

PROS	CONS
• Maintains a steady low temperature.	• Requires frequent monitoring of simmering water level to prevent burning.
• No need for extra gadgets.	

STOVE-TOP INDIRECT HEAT VIA MASON JAR

Add the cannabis and infusion medium to a quart-sized mason jar. Place a folded kitchen towel in the bottom of the pot to diffuse some of the heat, then place the mason jar on top of the towel. Add water to the pot as far as you can without the jar floating. Simmer for about 4 hours, adding water as needed.

PROS	CONS
• Maintains a steady low temperature. • No need for extra gadgets.	• Requires frequent monitoring of simmering water level to prevent burning.

INFUSION-MAKING TIPS

There are a number of things you can do to ensure the best results of your cannabis infusion cooking experiences:

- Stock up. Instead of having to plan well in advance each time you want to make edibles, keeping a stash of infused "staples" in your refrigerator or freezer allows you to create edibles on a whim.
- Be cautious with temperature. THC is completely burned off at 392°F, but starts to break down long before. Slow infusing over low temperatures yields the best results. Cooking in a slow cooker or in a double boiler ensures your infusion never gets too hot.
- When infusing with a double boiler, always cover the top pot to reduce the amount of evaporation.
- If infusing in a mason jar in simmering water, cover the jar, but "burp" (release the air inside) the jar every hour or so to relieve pressure buildup.
- For best flavor and texture, don't grind your weed into a fine powder. Crumble with your fingers or use a coarse grinder.
- Improve the flavor of edibles by making extra strong infusions, as this allows you to use less in the finished recipe and still get a proper dose.
- A French press coffeepot makes separating plant material from the infused medium quick and easy.
- You also can strain infusions over a cheesecloth-lined strainer into a clean container.

BYPASSING INFUSIONS WITH CONCENTRATES

While you can make infusions out of concentrates such as kief, hash, or hash oil, you can also bypass this step and stir the decarboxylated concentrate directly into recipes. This can save a lot of time and allows you to make a single dish with a small amount of concentrate, as opposed to needing a larger quantity of cannabis to make a batch of butter, oil, or other medium.

Cooking with concentrates lets you medicate all kinds of recipes without depending on a significant quantity of butter or oil to carry the medication. It also eliminates a lot of the green herbal flavor that most people don't like.

On the downside, concentrates can cost significantly more, especially hash oil. However, you can often find bargains on kief, or easily make it yourself with minimal time and investment. See the Resources section of this book for an instruction link.

BUYING PREMADE STAPLES

In states with robust dispensary systems in place, cannabis cooks can now choose to forgo making staples and enjoy the convenience of purchasing premade marijuana-infused butter, oil, and other staples.

PROS	CONS
• Convenient—just add to your recipe and go.	• Significantly more expensive than making your own.
• Usually lab tested for contents and dosing. Be sure to read the bottle to know how much THC you will be ingesting.	• Not always available.
• Eliminates the need to purchase cannabis for cooking.	
• Delivers consistent results batch after batch, if you purchase from a reputable manufacturer.	

VERDICT

If you enjoy using convenience foods, then premade staples are for you.

WHAT TO DO IF YOU ACCIDENTALLY CONSUME TOO MUCH MARIJUANA

Because it can take so long to feel the effects, there is no easier way to ingest too much marijuana than by eating it. People may eat some, think it's not working because it can take well over an hour to feel the effects, eat more, and inadvertently ingest too much.

The first thing to do if you or someone you know has consumed too much marijuana is to stay calm. It might be uncomfortable, but it is not dangerous and the side effects will pass in a few hours. There is no such thing as a fatal marijuana overdose. You will not stop breathing and your organs will not shut down. Cannabis simply does not work that way in the body.

Here's what to do if you ever feel too high:

Chew Peppercorns. Due to their similar terpenoid profiles and how the plants interact, black peppercorns can counteract high levels of THC. Try chewing on two or three peppercorns for a few minutes when feeling too high, and enjoy relief in minutes.

Consume CBDs. Cannabidiol can also counter the effects of too much THC. My favorite remedies are CBD breath sprays—a few spritzes and you will almost instantly feel yourself starting to come down—but CBD in any form will work.

Eat and Drink. Drink plenty of water and, unless you are feeling nauseous, get some nonmedicated foods in your system. Edibles are felt more profoundly on an empty stomach.

Sleep It Off. The best thing to do when you have ingested too much marijuana is go to bed and get some sleep.

DOSING

When it comes to the ideal cannabis edibles dose, everyone is different—and I mean *drastically* different. Five milligrams of THC will be too much for some folks, while 105 milligrams won't be enough for others. This is because everyone's cannabinoid needs vary, and a lot of complex factors come into play regarding how individuals respond to marijuana.

California and Colorado have put caps of 10 milligrams of THC per serving on commercial edibles. While this might be perfectly reasonable for some people, others will feel absolutely nothing from such a low dose. When it comes to cannabis edibles, the best way to get exactly what you need is to make them yourself.

THE TRUTH ABOUT DOSING

Just because a given recipe tells you to use a certain amount of cannabis does not mean it is going to deliver what YOU individually need, a reality which provides a continual source of frustration for home cooks.

For so long, home cooks used to pick a reasonable amount of marijuana to use based upon tolerance level and the strength of the plant material and hope for the best. It didn't always work so well. Some people made edibles far too strong for their tolerances, while others created foods that failed to deliver at all. Both scenarios waste weed.

Don't worry, I will teach you how to estimate the milligrams of THC per serving in your homemade edibles before you cook, so you'll always get what you need.

TESTING YOUR TOLERANCE

All the talk of per-serving milligram doses is great, but the numbers mean nothing if you don't know your personal tolerance level. Here's how to find yours.

If you live in an area where you can buy commercial edibles, choose a lab-tested brand with a reputation for consistency, such as Cheeba Chews or Kiva. Alternatively, you can use homemade edibles to test your tolerance level, but first you will need to do the calculations in this chapter.

Once you know the amount of THC in your food, begin by eating a 10-milligram dose. If you are brand-new to edibles or consider yourself a "lightweight," begin with a 5-milligram dose. Make a note of how you feel a few hours later. If you felt good, congratulations. You have found your ideal dose range. If not, try eating 5 or 10 milligrams more the next day. Continue increasing the milligram amount day after day until you find a dosage amount that makes you feel good. Keep in mind the point of the exercise is to find a comfortable therapeutic dose, not to get baked out of your mind.

If you don't know how strong a given batch of cannabis butter, oil, or other edible is, it's best to test the waters before chowing down with gusto. Start with a half portion, or even a quarter portion if you are sensitive to edibles. Wait at least three hours. If you feel the effects, don't eat any more. If you feel nothing, try another piece, or wait until the next day and try a larger portion. Even if you don't feel a "high," you will still be getting medicinal benefits.

THE HOMEMADE EDIBLES DOSING FORMULA

This four-step formula will give you as close an approximation as you can get in dosing homemade edibles without going to the expense of lab testing. If you are cooking with lab-tested cannabis, you can skip step 1 below and simply look on the label to find the percentage of THC.

STEP 1 ESTIMATE THE THC PERCENTAGE OF YOUR CANNABIS

A US government study from 2009 says that the national average marijuana contains 10 percent THC, so start your percentage estimate at 10 percent and adjust up or down from there, keeping in mind that all marijuana is *not* created equal. The government-grown cannabis from the University of Mississippi supplied to researchers tops out at 3 percent THC, whereas a 2015 Colorado study saw some top-shelf strains from that state come in at a whopping 30 percent THC.

The following will give you typical THC percentages you are likely to encounter:

3 to 5%: Government weed or low-quality "schwag"

5 to 10%: Higher potency brick weed

10 to 15%: Decent quality trim and shake, average homegrown cannabis, a majority of black-market marijuana

15 to 25%: Most decent-quality dispensary cannabis and better-quality black-market marijuana

Above 25%: If you're lucky enough to find this, don't waste it cooking—smoke it or vape it instead

STEP 2 CALCULATE THE AMOUNT OF THC IN YOUR CANNABIS

For this example, let's use cannabis that is 10 percent THC. As 1 gram equals 1000 milligrams, calculate how much THC is in 1 gram of our starting material by multiplying the percentage of THC (.10 in this case) by 1000. So .10 × 1000 equals 100 milligrams THC per gram in our starting plant material.

STEP 3 CALCULATE THE AMOUNT OF THC IN YOUR HOMEMADE INFUSIONS/STAPLES

To do this you need to decide how much cannabis you are going to use, and how much butter or oil (or other ingredient) you are going to infuse.

For this example, I will use the same amounts I used to create all the recipes in this book: ½ ounce (14 grams) of marijuana to make 1 cup (8 ounces) of cannabutter or Cannabis Butter (page 37). Multiply the 14 grams of starting material by the 100 milligrams of THC per gram as determined in step 2 (14 × 100) and see that our 1 cup of infused butter contains 1400 milligrams of THC.

To calculate how much THC is in each ounce of butter, we divide 1400 milligrams of THC by the 8 ounces (1 cup) of butter, which gives us 175 milligrams of THC per 1 ounce of infused butter. Are you with me so far?

STEP 4 CALCULATE THE AMOUNT OF THC PER SERVING IN YOUR HOMEMADE EDIBLES

This calculation determines the THC dosage in each serving of your finished recipe. To do this you will need to know how much of your infusion you will use in the recipe and how many servings the recipe makes.

Let's say you are going to use ½ cup (4 ounces) of cannabutter to make 36 cookies. You already know the cannabutter contains 175 milligrams per ounce, so there will be 700 milligrams in the entire recipe (4 × 175). Now all you have to do is divide the total amount of THC (700 milligrams) in the recipe by the number of servings (36) the recipe makes, and you will see that each cookie will contain about 19 milligrams of THC.

If 19 milligrams THC was more than you wanted, you could cut the amount of cannabutter in the recipe and make up the difference in unmedicated butter. Conversely, if you want stronger cookies, you might opt to dissolve some decarboxylated kief or hash into your cannabutter by gently heating them together. This is how to play with recipes in order to get the exact dosage you want.

CALCULATING DOSAGES WITH CONCENTRATES

If you are using concentrates, the process and calculations are the same, but what changes is the percentage of THC and the amounts you will typically use. In the absence of lab tests, check the potency of what you are using by smoking or vaping a little and estimate accordingly. Start your estimate in the middle range and adjust up or down depending on quality:

- The THC percentage for kief and water, or bubble hash, will weigh in between 30 to 50 percent, and in rare cases of exceptionally good product you might find 60 percent.
- For CO_2 or butane hash oils, the typical range is 50 to 70 percent, with exceptional product going up to 80 percent.

CALCULATING DOSAGES WITH STORE-BOUGHT STAPLES

When using store-bought staples, use the label to determine how many milligrams of THC are in the amount of infusion used in your recipe, then divide by the number of servings in the recipe.

DOSAGE CALCULATION TIPS AND TROUBLESHOOTING

Here are some tips:

- For your convenience, I have created a free online dosage calculator that does all the math and metric conversions for you. Find it at: bit.ly/dosingcalculator.
- It is not possible to predict CBD or other cannabinoid percentages without lab testing. If you are using lab-tested cannabis, you can use this formula to estimate the amount of any cannabinoid tested for.
- Even with decarboxylation, you might not convert 100 percent of the THCa to psychoactive THC, so it is best to estimate slightly less than the actual calculation.

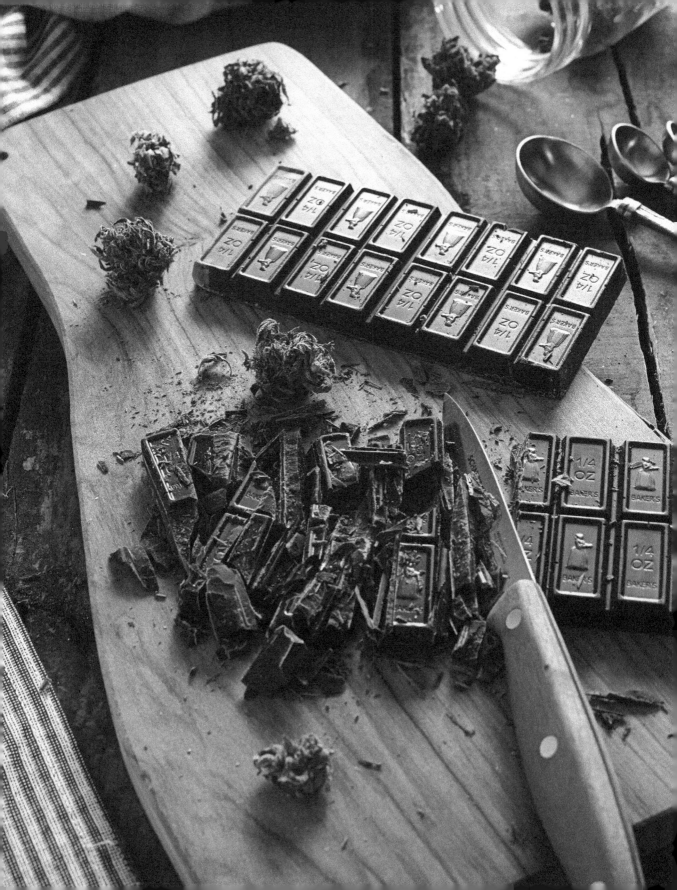

PART 2
EVERYDAY RECIPES

Cooking with marijuana requires no exotic or expensive devices, just the few basic tools you already have, some marijuana, and a little bit of knowledge. If you lack the latter, you have come to the right place, as *The Easy Cannabis Cookbook* will show you just how accessible cooking with marijuana can be.

This second part of the book is filled with tempting, tested recipes that incorporate cannabis. Though you will find some dessert recipes, I have also included formulas for making all kinds of other foods like breakfasts, soups, salads, snacks, and main courses. The sooner the general public stops thinking of edible marijuana as an excuse for a brownie and treats it like any other food, the healthier we all will be.

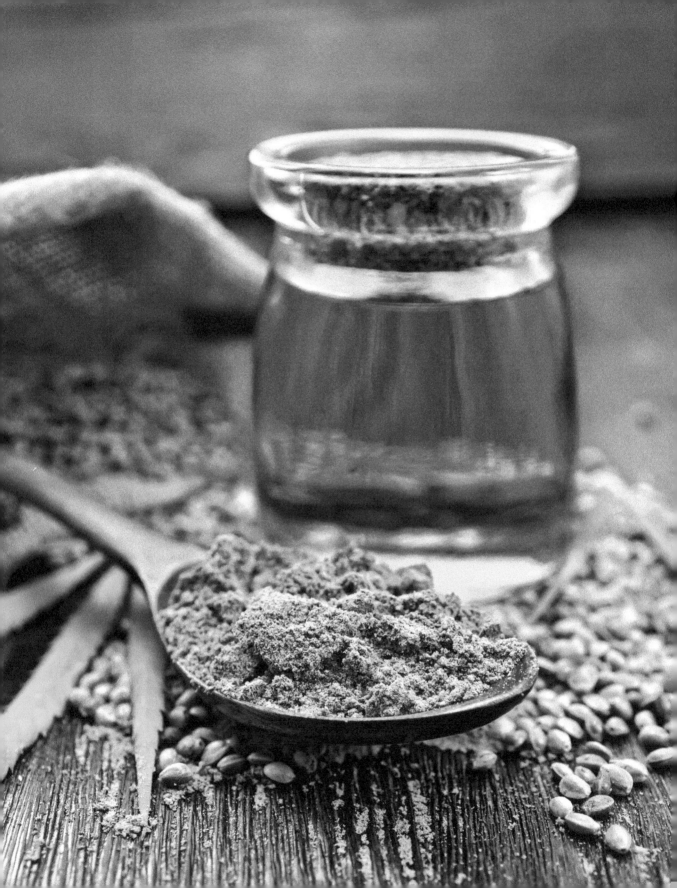

CHAPTER 4
STAPLES

The cannabis staples in this section are dosed based on using cannabis with 10 percent THC, the national average. If you are cooking with cannabis that is more or less than 10 percent, refer to chapter 3 and adjust the dosage accordingly based on your revised calculations.

Regardless of the THC percentage, you can make any of these infusions stronger or weaker by adding more or less marijuana. Once again, the dosing formula in chapter 3 is your key to customization.

If you use the slow-cooker method, you can set it and forget once you stir together the cannabis and liquid.

Before storing, label each of your infusions with the per-ounce THC content so it's easy to figure out the per-serving doses for the recipes you make with them.

DRAINING AND STRAINING

Unless otherwise noted, these instructions apply to all the recipes in this chapter.

- Place a cheesecloth-lined strainer over a large pot or bowl and strain the liquid infusion. Once it is cool enough to handle, squeeze out as much liquid as possible from the cheesecloth and discard the plant material.

- Alternatively, pour the liquid infusion and plant material in a large French press coffeepot, plunge to separate, then pour out the liquid. Discard the plant material.
- You can optionally strain the liquid one more time to get rid of any fine sediment. Place a double layer of cheesecloth over a strainer and pour the liquid infusion through. Alternatively, a fine-mesh yogurt strainer makes quick work of straining sediment, too.

CANNABIS BUTTER
VEGETARIAN, GLUTEN-FREE, NUT-FREE

MAKES 1 CUP

PREP TIME:
5 MINUTES

INFUSE TIME:
4 TO 6 HOURS

Cannabutter is one of the cannabis cook's best friends. You'll use it for most of the baking you do and in lots of other recipes. For best results and maximum versatility, use unsalted butter.

DOSAGE WHEN MADE WITH 10% THC CANNABIS: ABOUT 175 MG THC PER OUNCE

1¼ cups butter
½ ounce crumbled decarboxylated cannabis

TO MAKE IN A SLOW COOKER

Add the butter and cannabis to the slow cooker, cover, and cook on low for 4 to 6 hours, stirring occasionally if desired.*

TO MAKE IN A DOUBLE BOILER

Add the butter and cannabis to the top of a double boiler and cook over simmering water for about 4 hours. Check the water level frequently and add more as necessary to keep several inches of simmering water in the lower pot. Stir the butter occasionally.*

TO MAKE IN A MASON JAR

1. Bring a saucepan of water to a simmer and place a clean, folded kitchen towel in the bottom of the pan.

2. Put the butter and cannabis in a mason jar and cover with the lid.

3. Place the jar on the towel in the simmering water for about 4 hours. Check the water level frequently and add more as necessary. Stir the butter occasionally. Open the jar every hour or so while infusing in order to relieve any pressure buildup.*

* Drain and strain the butter as outlined in the general instructions at the beginning of this chapter. Label and store in an airtight container in the refrigerator for up to 1 month.

Storage tip For longer storage, put in an airtight plastic container and freeze, then remove just the amount you need to cook with. Fats can go rancid even in the freezer, so use within 6 months.

CANNABIS OIL
NUT-FREE, VEGETARIAN, GLUTEN-FREE, DAIRY-FREE

MAKES 1 CUP

—

PREP TIME:
5 MINUTES

—

INFUSE TIME:
4 TO 6 HOURS

You can infuse any type of edible oil, so use whatever works best for the recipes you plan to cook. I try to keep a variety of infused oils on hand. Vegetable, olive, and coconut oil will cover most recipes you'll want to make.

DOSAGE WHEN MADE WITH 10% THC CANNABIS: ABOUT 175 MG THC PER OUNCE

1¼ cups edible oil of your choice
½ ounce crumbled decarboxylated cannabis

TO MAKE IN A SLOW COOKER

Add the oil and cannabis to the slow cooker, cover, and cook on low for 4 to 6 hours, stirring occasionally if desired.*

TO MAKE IN A DOUBLE BOILER

Add the oil and cannabis to the top of a double boiler and cook over simmering water for about 4 hours. Check the water level frequently and add more as necessary to keep several inches of simmering water in the lower pot. Stir the water occasionally.*

TO MAKE IN A MASON JAR

1. Bring a saucepan of water to a simmer and place a clean, folded kitchen towel in the bottom of the pan.

2. Put the oil and cannabis in a mason jar and cover with the lid.

3. Place the jar on the towel in the simmering water for about 4 hours. Check the water level frequently and add more as necessary. Stir the oil occasionally. Open the jar every hour or so while infusing in order to relieve any pressure buildup.*

* Drain and strain the oil as outlined in the general instructions at the beginning of this chapter. Label and store in a glass jar with an airtight lid.

Storage Tip I find it handy to freeze medicated oils and butter in ice-cube trays to make it easy to remove just a small amount.

CANNABIS MILK OR CREAM
VEGETARIAN, GLUTEN-FREE, NUT-FREE

MAKES 1 CUP

--

PREP TIME:
5 MINUTES

--

INFUSE TIME:
1 TO 1½ HOURS

Dairy products can curdle when exposed to too much heat and ultra-long cooking times, which is why I prefer the double-boiler or mason-jar technique for this infusion. Infused dairy products are handy not only for recipes, but also to quickly medicate drinks like coffee, tea, or hot cocoa.

DOSAGE WHEN MADE WITH 10% THC MARIJUANA: ABOUT 175 MG THC PER OUNCE

1¼ **cups whole milk or heavy (whipping) cream**
½ **ounce crumbled decarboxylated cannabis**

TO MAKE IN A DOUBLE BOILER

Add the milk or cream and cannabis to the top of a double boiler and cook over simmering water for about 1 hour. Check the water level frequently and add more as necessary to keep several inches of simmering water in the lower pot. Stir the milk occasionally.*

TO MAKE IN A MASON JAR

1. Bring a saucepan of water to a simmer and place a clean, folded kitchen towel in the bottom of the pan.

2. Put the milk or cream and cannabis in a mason jar and cover with the lid.

3. Place the jar on the towel in the simmering water for about 1½ hours. Check the water level frequently and add more as necessary. Stir the milk occasionally. Open the jar every hour or so while infusing in order to relieve any pressure buildup.*

* Drain and strain as outlined in the general instructions at the beginning of this chapter. The length of time milk or cream will stay fresh in the fridge depends on how fresh the milk was to begin with. It's usually safe for 3 to 5 days or until the milk begins to sour. Label and store in an airtight container.

Variation tip You can also infuse half-and-half as well as vegan milks, such as almond, soy, or coconut milk, using these same instructions. THC binds best in the presence of fat, so avoid fat-free products.

CANNABIS HONEY OR SYRUP
VEGETARIAN, GLUTEN-FREE, DAIRY-FREE, NUT-FREE

MAKES 1 CUP

PREP TIME:
10 MINUTES

INFUSE TIME:
6 TO 8 HOURS

These instructions work for any sticky, syrupy substance, such as honey, maple syrup, agave sweetener, corn syrup, or molasses. Since the cannabis is placed in a cheesecloth bundle during the infusion process (which makes cleanup far easier), less cannabis is used, so it's best to give these staples a bit more time to infuse. It's also a good idea to stir more frequently.

DOSAGE WHEN MADE WITH 10% THC CANNABIS: ABOUT 85 MG THC PER OUNCE

¼ **ounce crumbled decarboxylated cannabis**
1⅛ **cups honey, agave sweetener, maple syrup, corn syrup, or molasses**

Cut a 10-by-10-inch piece of cheesecloth and place the cannabis in the center of it. Gather the cheesecloth corners together and tightly tie with kitchen twine to make a bundle.

TO MAKE IN A SLOW COOKER
Add the honey to the slow cooker along with the cannabis bundle, cover, and cook on low for 6 to 8 hours, stirring every hour or two to move the bundle around.*

TO MAKE IN A DOUBLE BOILER
Add the honey and cannabis bundle to the top of a double boiler and cook over simmering water for about 6 hours. Check the water level frequently and add more as necessary to keep several inches of simmering water in the lower pot. Stir the honey occasionally.*

TO MAKE IN A MASON JAR
1. Bring a saucepan of water to a simmer and place a clean, folded kitchen towel in the bottom of the pan.

2. Put the honey and cannabis bundle in a mason jar and cover with the lid.

3. Place the jar on the towel in the simmering water for about 6 hours. Check the water level frequently and add more as necessary. Stir the honey occasionally. Open the jar every hour or so while infusing in order to relieve any pressure buildup.*

* To drain, cool until the bundle can be safely handled, then squeeze out as much honey as possible. Discard the bundle. Label and store the honey in an airtight jar in the refrigerator for up to 6 months.

Ingredient tip For a healthy way to use up every last drop of infused sweetness, after squeezing out as much honey or syrup as you can from the cannabis bundle, drop the bundle in a teapot with a few tea bags and pour boiling water over it. Steep for a few minutes, then strain into cups for a delicious, medicated tea.

CANNABIS SIMPLE SYRUP
VEGAN, GLUTEN-FREE, DAIRY-FREE, NUT-FREE

MAKES 1 CUP

PREP TIME:
5 MINUTES

INFUSE TIME:
1½ TO 6 HOURS

This version of the bartender's staple is a great way to simultaneously sweeten and medicate cold drinks—think iced tea and iced coffee drinks, summer fruit punches, Mexican-style *aguas frescas*, and more. Edibles are all about refreshing, restoring, and healing, and this simple syrup offers an easy path to relief.

DOSAGE WHEN MADE WITH 10% THC CANNABIS: ABOUT 85 MG THC PER OUNCE

1¼ cups water
1¼ cups granulated sugar
¼ ounce crumbled decarboxylated cannabis

TO MAKE IN A SLOW COOKER

Add the water, sugar, and cannabis to the slow cooker, cover, and cook on low for about 2 hours, stirring occasionally if desired.*

TO MAKE IN A DOUBLE BOILER

Add the water, sugar, and cannabis to the top of a double boiler and cook over simmering water for about 1½ hours. Check the water level frequently and add more as necessary to keep several inches of simmering water in the lower pot. Stir the syrup occasionally.*

TO MAKE IN A MASON JAR

1. Bring a saucepan of water to a simmer and place a clean, folded kitchen towel in the bottom of the pan.

2. Put the water, sugar, and cannabis in a mason jar and cover with the lid.

3. Place the jar on the towel in the simmering water for about 6 hours. Check the water level frequently and add more as necessary. Stir the syrup occasionally. Open the jar every hour or so while infusing in order to relieve any pressure buildup.*

* Drain and strain as outlined in the general instructions at the beginning of this chapter. Label and store in an airtight container in the refrigerator for about 6 months.

Variation tip Add a handful of other flavorful herbs to your infusion to make gourmet drinks like mint iced tea or lavender lemonade.

CANNABIS TINCTURE
VEGAN, GLUTEN-FREE, DAIRY-FREE, NUT-FREE

Alcohol-based tinctures could not be easier to make or use to medicate most any recipe—just stir in a few drops. Besides enhancing edibles, tinctures are also effective when taken sublingually. Place a few drops under your tongue and feel the effects far faster than waiting for an edible to digest.

DOSAGE WHEN MADE WITH 10% THC CANNABIS: ABOUT 175 MG THC PER OUNCE

1⅛ cups high-proof alcohol, such as Everclear, 151 rum, or high-proof vodka

½ ounce crumbled decarboxylated cannabis

1. Put the alcohol and cannabis in a mason jar. Cover tightly and shake. Store in a cool, dark cabinet and let steep for 4 days, taking the jar out to shake each day.

2. Strain by pouring through a cheesecloth-lined strainer or through a fine-mesh yogurt strainer. Label and store in an airtight, dark glass bottle in the fridge. Tinctures will keep almost indefinitely.

Variation tip You can substitute other alcohols like tequila, whiskey, or bourbon, but generally speaking, the higher the proof, the better your tincture will infuse. For lighter dosed, infused alcohols to use in cocktails, increase the amount of spirits in this recipe to 4 cups.

CANNABIS SUGAR
VEGAN, GLUTEN-FREE, DAIRY-FREE, NUT-FREE

In addition to endless uses in all kinds of recipes, medicated granulated sugar offers a discreet way to add a little cannabis to coffee, tea, cereal, or anything else you'd sprinkle sugar in. Like the other infusions, it's easy to make and keep on hand so you never need to be without a quick medicating dose when you need it most.

DOSAGE WHEN MADE WITH CANNABIS TINCTURE (PAGE 42), 175 MG THC PER CUP

1 cup granulated sugar
2 tablespoons Cannabis Tincture (page 42) made with Everclear

1. Preheat the oven to 200°F.

2. Put the sugar and Cannabis Tincture in a small bowl and mix thoroughly. The mixture will be a bit grainy.

3. Spread sugar in a thin layer on a baking sheet. Bake for 1 hour, removing the pan to stir the sugar every 15 minutes. The sugar will have a dry consistency with all the alcohol evaporated when it is done.

4. Let it cool. If the sugar has lumps, run it through a blender or food processor, or alternately press the sugar through a sieve to restore its normal texture. Store in an airtight container at room temperature. It will keep indefinitely as long as it doesn't accumulate any moisture, in which case it will turn gummy.

Ingredient tip It's important to use tincture made from Everclear or another extremely high-proof alcohol when making Cannabis Sugar. Lower proof alcohols contain too much water, which can make the mixture a gummy mess.

MARIJUANA MAYONNAISE
VEGETARIAN, GLUTEN-FREE, DAIRY-FREE, NUT-FREE

MAKES ¾ CUP
1 TBSP = 1 SERV
—
PREP TIME:
5 MINUTES

With a blender or food processor, you can make homemade mayonnaise in just minutes. This version is so easy to whip up and superior in taste to store-bought mayo, you'll never need to buy it again. If you have infused oil on hand, it takes no extra time to make it medicated.

DOSAGE WHEN MADE WITH CANNABIS OIL (PAGE 38): ABOUT 25 MG PER TABLESPOON

2 egg yolks
4 teaspoons freshly squeezed lemon juice
1 teaspoon Dijon mustard
¾ cup vegetable oil
¼ cup Cannabis Oil (page 38)
Salt
Freshly ground black pepper

1. Put the egg yolks, lemon juice, and mustard in a food processor or blender and process until well combined.

2. With the machine running, drizzle in the vegetable oil and Cannabis Oil in a slow, steady stream. The mixture will thicken as it emulsifies but will not be quite as thick as commercial mayonnaise.

3. Season with salt and pepper. Refrigerate in an airtight container, and use within 2 days.

Ingredient tip Look for pasteurized eggs to avoid possible foodborne illness in raw eggs, especially if you have a compromised immune system.

CANNABIS PESTO
VEGETARIAN, GLUTEN-FREE

MAKES 1 CUP
2 TBSP = 1 SERV

PREP TIME:
10 MINUTES

Serve this versatile, cannabis-fortified pesto sauce with pasta, or over steamed or grilled vegetables, chicken, fish, or tofu for an instant meal. You can even use a light coating of pesto instead of sauce on pizza.

DOSAGE WHEN MADE WITH CANNABIS OIL (PAGE 38): ABOUT 20 MG PER 2 TABLESPOONS

1 cup loosely packed fresh basil

½ cup freshly grated Parmesan cheese

¼ cup toasted pine nuts or walnuts

¾ teaspoon minced garlic

¼ cup plus 2 tablespoons extra-virgin olive oil

2 tablespoons Cannabis Olive Oil (page 38)

Salt

Freshly ground black pepper

Add the basil, Parmesan, nuts, and garlic to a food processor or blender. Process to mix. With the machine running, drizzle in the olive oil and Cannabis Oil in a slow, steady stream. Season with salt and pepper. Refrigerate in an airtight container for up to 5 days or freeze for up to 1 month.

Storage tip Freeze extra pesto sauce in ice-cube trays, then transfer the frozen pesto cubes to plastic freezer bags for longer storage. When ready to use in cooking, simply remove the amount you need.

CANNABIS VINAIGRETTE
VEGETARIAN, GLUTEN-FREE

MAKES 1 CUP
1 TBSP = 1 SERV

—

**PREP TIME:
10 MINUTES**

Vinaigrettes, mixtures of seasoned oil and vinegar or citrus juice, are easy ways to use cannabis-infused oil. The flavor possibilities are endless when you try different ingredient combinations. Discover the versatility of vinaigrettes as salad dressings, or add a dash of flavor and medication to steamed or grilled veggies, fish, poultry, or meats.

DOSAGE WHEN MADE WITH CANNABIS OIL (PAGE 38): ABOUT 20 MG PER TABLESPOON

FOR A BASIC MEDICATED VINAIGRETTE

- ½ **cup extra-virgin olive oil or vegetable oil**
- ¼ **cup Cannabis Oil (page 38)**
- ¼ **cup vinegar or other acid, such as freshly squeezed lemon or lime juice**
- **Flavoring ingredients, such as mustard, soy sauce, hot sauce, Worcestershire sauce, sesame oil, walnut oil, grated ginger, citrus zest, or grated cheese**
- **A touch of sweetness to bring out flavor, such as sugar, honey, agave, or maple syrup**
- **Herbs, spices, salt, and freshly ground pepper**

Whisk together all the ingredients or combine in a blender or food processor until emulsified. Refrigerate in an airtight container for up to 5 days. Always shake the container before using.

Variation tip Try countless vinai-grette variations by changing the types of oils, vinegars or other acidic ingredients, and seasonings. Three of my favorites are featured on the next page.

ITALIAN PARMESAN VINAIGRETTE

¾ cup extra-virgin olive oil
¼ cup Cannabis Olive Oil (page 38)
¼ cup red wine vinegar
2 tablespoons grated
   Parmesan cheese
2 teaspoons Dijon mustard
1 teaspoon minced garlic
1 teaspoon dried parsley
¼ teaspoon sugar
Salt
Freshly ground black pepper

ASIAN VINAIGRETTE

½ cup vegetable oil
¼ cup Cannabis Vegetable Oil
   (page 38)
¼ cup rice vinegar
1 tablespoon minced ginger
2 teaspoons toasted sesame oil
2 teaspoons soy sauce
2 teaspoons honey or agave
1 teaspoon minced garlic

LEMON VINAIGRETTE

¾ cup extra-virgin olive oil
¼ cup Cannabis Olive Oil (page 38)
¼ cup freshly squeezed lemon juice
1 teaspoon minced garlic
1 teaspoon dried oregano
¼ teaspoon sugar

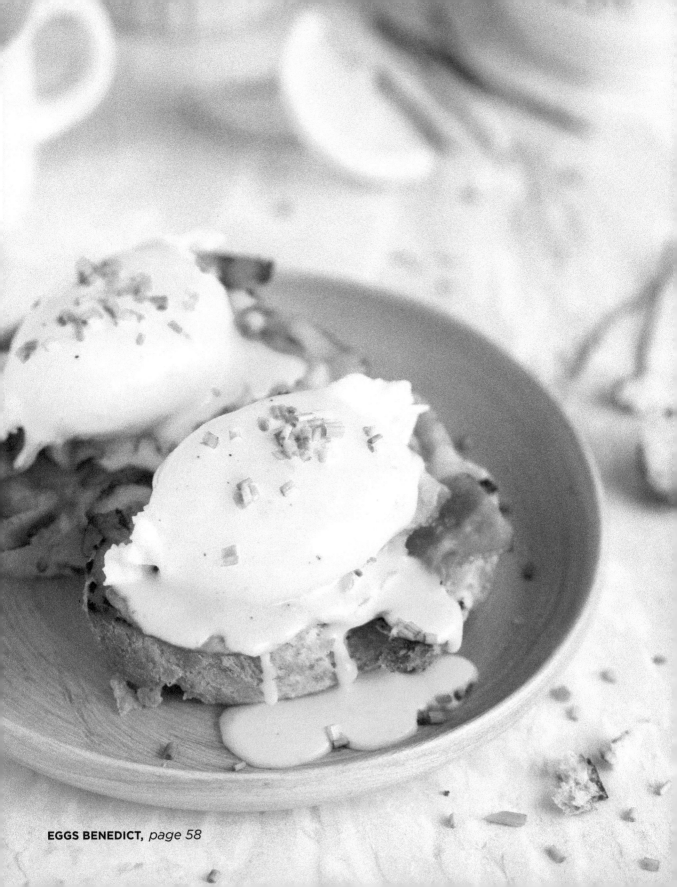

EGGS BENEDICT, *page 58*

CHAPTER 5
BREAKFAST

MAKES 3 CUPS
½ CUP = 1 SERV
—
PREP TIME:
10 MINUTES
—
BAKE TIME:
35 MINUTES

CRANBERRY HEMP SEED GRANOLA

VEGETARIAN, GLUTEN-FREE, DAIRY-FREE

Making homemade granola is so quick and easy, you'll never be tempted to buy store-bought versions again. I prefer using infused coconut oil in this recipe for the fabulous flavor it adds, but any infused edible oil will work in its place.

DOSAGE WHEN MADE WITH CANNABIS OIL (PAGE 38): ABOUT 25 MG THC PER SERVING

1½ **cups rolled oats**
¾ **cup dried cranberries**
⅓ **cup sliced almonds**
⅓ **cup sweetened coconut flakes**
¼ **cup hulled hemp seeds**
¼ **cup honey**
⅛ **cup Cannabis Oil (page 38),
    melted if using coconut oil**
⅛ **cup coconut oil, melted,
    or other oil**
1 **egg white**
¼ **teaspoon cinnamon**
⅛ **teaspoon salt**

1. Preheat the oven to 300°F. Line a large baking sheet with parchment paper.

2. In a large bowl, mix together the oats, cranberries, almonds, coconut flakes, and hemp seeds.

3. In a small bowl, whisk together the honey, Cannabis Oil, coconut oil, egg white, cinnamon, and salt. Pour this mixture over the oat mixture and stir until well combined.

4. Spread the oat mixture in a thin, even layer on the prepared baking sheet. Bake for about 35 minutes or until browned to your liking, stirring the granola every 10 minutes or so during baking.

5. Let cool and store in an airtight container for up to 2 weeks or more (if you can resist temptation and make it last that long).

Ingredient Tip Hemp seeds contain almost no THC but are fiber-rich nutritional powerhouses containing high levels of omega-3 and omega-6 fatty acids, proteins, and minerals.

BANANA BREAD
VEGETARIAN, NUT-FREE

MAKES 7 MINI LOAVES
½ LOAF = 1 SERV
--
PREP TIME: 10 MINUTES
--
BAKE TIME: 25 MINUTES

Sweet bananas make a casual anytime cake that needs no frosting. The trick is that the bananas need to be very, very ripe so they can be mashed until smooth. Bananas become sweeter the longer they ripen.

DOSAGE WHEN MADE WITH CANNABIS BUTTER (PAGE 37): ABOUT 25 MG THC PER SERVING

Vegetable shortening or nonstick cooking spray
¾ cup all-purpose flour
½ cup whole-wheat flour
¼ cup sugar
¼ cup packed brown sugar
½ teaspoon salt
½ teaspoon baking powder
½ teaspoon baking soda
½ teaspoon nutmeg
1½ cups mashed bananas (about 4 medium bananas)
¼ cup buttermilk
¼ cup Cannabis Butter (page 37), at room temperature
2 tablespoons honey
1 large egg
1 teaspoon vanilla extract

1. Preheat the oven to 350°F. Grease 7 (2¾-by-3¾-inch) mini-loaf pans with the vegetable shortening or nonstick cooking spray.

2. In a medium bowl, combine the all-purpose flour, whole-wheat flour, sugar, brown sugar, salt, baking powder, baking soda, and nutmeg and stir to mix.

3. In a large bowl, combine the mashed bananas, buttermilk, Cannabis Butter, honey, egg, and vanilla extract and beat well with an electric mixer or by hand.

4. Add the dry ingredients to the large bowl and mix until just combined. Do not overmix.

5. Fill the loaf pans slightly more than half full.

6. Bake until a toothpick inserted into the center of the loaf comes out clean, 20 to 25 minutes.

Continued

7. Cool the loaves in the pans on a wire rack for about 10 minutes before removing them to finish cooling on the wire rack. Serve warm or at room temperature. Individually wrap the loaves in plastic wrap, and they will keep for about 3 days, or they can be frozen for several months.

Variation tip Mix and match 1 cup of any of these into the batter for a flavor boost: toasted nuts, sweetened dried cranberries, fresh blueberries, raisins, chocolate chips, white chocolate chips, peanut butter chips.

CARROT RAISIN BRAN MUFFINS

VEGETARIAN

MAKES 12 MUFFINS
1 MUFFIN = 1 SERV
—
PREP TIME: 15 MINUTES
—
BAKE TIME: 25 MINUTES

Sweet carrots and raisins combine with nutty bran flakes to make these hearty, healthy muffins. It's important to use a neutral oil like vegetable oil with this recipe—or any quick bread—so as not to dull the flavors. Nut oils will overpower the other ingredients.

DOSAGE WHEN MADE WITH CANNABIS OIL (PAGE 38): ABOUT 25 MG THC PER SERVING

1 cup milk
1 cup shredded carrots
¼ cup Cannabis Vegetable Oil (page 38)
¼ cup vegetable oil
1 egg
2 teaspoons finely grated orange zest
1½ cups crushed raisin bran flake cereal
1½ cups all-purpose flour
⅓ cup sugar
⅓ cup firmly packed brown sugar
1 tablespoon baking powder
2 teaspoons pumpkin pie spice
½ teaspoon salt
1 cup raisins
¾ cup chopped walnuts or pecans (optional)

1. Preheat the oven to 375°F. Place paper liners in 12 regular-size muffin cups.

2. In a medium bowl, whisk together the milk, carrots, Cannabis Oil, vegetable oil, egg, and orange zest until combined.

3. In a large bowl, combine the bran flakes, flour, sugar, brown sugar, baking powder, pumpkin pie spice, and salt.

4. Add the wet ingredients to the dry and stir just until all the flour is moistened. The batter will be lumpy.

5. Stir in the raisins and walnuts (if using).

6. Spoon the batter into the prepared muffin cups, filling each about three-quarters full.

Continued

7. Bake until the muffin tops have browned and a toothpick inserted into the center comes out clean, about 25 minutes. Serve warm, or cool to room temperature on a wire rack. Store the muffins in an airtight container at room temperature for about 3 days.

Storage Tip Like most muffins and quick breads, this recipe freezes well. Individually wrap the muffins in plastic wrap, stack them between layers of waxed paper, and store in zip-top plastic freezer bags. Thaw at room temperature and enjoy.

DUTCH BABY PANCAKE
VEGETARIAN, NUT-FREE

SERVES 2

--

PREP TIME:
5 MINUTES

--

BAKE TIME:
25 MINUTES

This fluffy baked pancake is certain to receive oohs and aahs when you remove it from the oven—and your guests never need to know how easy it is to make. Of course, when serving an edible to someone else, always get their permission and inform them of the dosage level.

DOSAGE WHEN MADE WITH CANNABIS MILK OR CREAM (PAGE 39): ABOUT 40 MG THC PER SERVING

¾ **cup milk**

¾ **cup all-purpose flour**

3 **eggs**

1 **tablespoon Cannabis Milk, Cream, or Half-and-Half (page 39)**

1 **tablespoon sugar**

½ **teaspoon salt**

⅛ **teaspoon ground nutmeg (optional)**

¼ **cup unsalted butter**

Juice of ½ lemon

2 **tablespoons confectioners' sugar**

1. Preheat the oven to 425°F.

2. In a large bowl, whisk together the milk, flour, eggs, Cannabis Milk, sugar, salt, and nutmeg (if using) until well combined and lump free.

3. Melt the butter in a large, preferably cast iron, skillet over medium heat. As soon as the butter is melted, pour the batter into the pan. Transfer the skillet to the oven and bake for about 20 minutes or until the pancake is puffed and golden brown. Lower the oven temperature to 300°F and continue baking for 5 more minutes.

4. Remove from the oven, sprinkle with the lemon juice and confectioners' sugar, and serve immediately.

Variation tip To make an apple Dutch Baby Pancake, peel and dice 1 apple and toss it with 1 tablespoon of sugar and ½ teaspoon of cinnamon. Prior to step 3, sauté the sugared apples in 1 tablespoon of unsalted butter over medium-high heat until slightly softened, about 5 minutes. Transfer the apples to a plate and wipe out the pan. Melt the butter as in step 3, return the apples to a small pile in the center of the skillet, pour the batter around the apples, and bake as directed in step 3.

MINI BACON, EGG, AND CHEESE QUICHES

NUT-FREE

MAKES 24 MINI QUICHES

—

PREP TIME:
20 MINUTES, PLUS
30 MINUTES TO CHILL

—

BAKE TIME: 40 MINUTES

Mini muffin pans make it easy to create delicious, bite-size quiches, so you can eat as many as your dosage needs merit. While I make this recipe with classic breakfast flavors, feel free to play with it and add your favorite omelet ingredients in place of (or in addition to) the bacon.

DOSAGE WHEN MADE WITH CANNABIS MILK (PAGE 39): ABOUT 15 MG THC PER MINI QUICHE

Nonstick cooking spray or vegetable shortening
¾ cup all-purpose flour
2 tablespoons unsalted butter
2 tablespoons vegetable shortening
4 tablespoons milk
½ cup cooked bacon bits
¾ cup shredded Swiss or Cheddar cheese
2 eggs
½ cup half-and-half
¼ cup Cannabis Half-and-Half (page 39)
¼ teaspoon salt
¼ teaspoon freshly ground black pepper

1. Preheat the oven to 375°F. Grease each muffin cup with the nonstick cooking spray or vegetable shortening.

2. To make the crust, add the flour, butter, and shortening to a food processor and pulse it 8 to 10 times to cut the butter into the flour until well combined.

3. Transfer this mixture from the processor to a large bowl and stir in the milk until the dough just holds together. Gather it into a ball, flatten it into a disc, wrap tightly in plastic wrap, and refrigerate for at least 30 minutes.

4. Lightly flour a clean surface and use a rolling pin to roll out the crust to ⅛-inch thickness. Use a 2½-inch round cookie cutter or a small glass with an opening that size to cut 24 circles from the dough, rerolling the dough as necessary.

5. Gently press each dough circle into a mini muffin cup. The dough should cover bottom and sides of the cup with no overhang.

6. Sprinkle about ½ teaspoon of bacon bits into each dough-lined cup.

7. Sprinkle about ¾ teaspoon of shredded cheese into each cup on top of the bacon.

8. In a medium bowl, whisk together the eggs, half-and-half, Cannabis Half-and-Half, salt, and pepper until well combined. Pour the egg mixture into each muffin cup until just filled.

9. Bake for about 40 minutes or until the quiches are set and the tops are golden brown. Cool in the pan for 5 minutes before removing the quiches. Serve hot, warm, at room temperature, or even cold.

Storage tip Stack cooled mini quiches between waxed paper in a large, airtight plastic container and freeze. Microwave 3 frozen mini quiches for about 40 seconds or heat in a 375°F oven for 35 to 40 minutes for a quick, medicated breakfast on the go.

EGGS BENEDICT
NUT-FREE

SERVES 2
--
PREP TIME:
15 MINUTES
--
COOK TIME:
5 MINUTES

Everyone's favorite indulgent brunch item sounds fancy, but this recipe proves it's not difficult to make. You can use the versatile, cannabis-enhanced hollandaise sauce from this recipe for lots of other foods, too. Try it on steamed, poached, or grilled fish dishes or steamed veggies.

DOSAGE WHEN MADE WITH CANNABIS BUTTER (PAGE 37): ABOUT 40 MG THC PER SERVING

FOR THE HOLLANDAISE SAUCE

⅓ **cup unsalted butter**
1 tablespoon Cannabis Butter (page 37)
3 egg yolks
2 tablespoons freshly squeezed lemon juice
¼ **teaspoon salt**
¼ **teaspoon freshly ground black pepper**
⅛ **teaspoon cayenne pepper**

FOR THE EGGS

1 teaspoon white vinegar
2 English muffins, halved
4 eggs
4 slices Canadian bacon
Chopped fresh Italian parsley

TO MAKE THE HOLLANDAISE SAUCE

1. In a small saucepan, melt the butter and Cannabis Butter together over medium-low heat just until bubbly. Do not let it brown.

2. Put the egg yolks, lemon juice, salt, pepper, and cayenne in the food processor and process at high speed for 2 to 3 seconds. With the machine running, drizzle in the melted butter in a slow, steady, thin stream until it is fully incorporated and the sauce is emulsified. Set aside.

TO MAKE THE EGGS

1. Fill a large skillet with about 3 inches of water and the vinegar and bring to a simmer.

2. Put the English muffins in a toaster to toast.

3. Carefully break an egg in a small ramekin or cup. Slip the egg into the simmering water. Quickly repeat this step with the 3 remaining eggs. Cook until the whites are set but the yolks are still soft, 2 to 3 minutes.

4. Place 2 toasted muffin halves on each of 2 plates. Top each muffin half with a slice of Canadian bacon. Use a slotted spoon to carefully remove each egg from the pan, letting any excess water drip off before placing 1 poached egg on top of each muffin half. Spoon the hollandaise sauce over the 4 muffin halves. Garnish each egg with the parsley. Serve immediately.

Storage Tip Store leftover hollandaise sauce in an airtight container in the refrigerator for up 3 days. Reheat it in the top of a double boiler, stirring constantly, until just heated. This is a delicate sauce that will break down in the microwave or over direct heat.

EGG SALAD SANDWICH

VEGETARIAN, DAIRY-FREE, NUT-FREE

MAKES 4
SANDWICHES
--
PREP TIME:
15 MINUTES

I love using green olives in this recipe as their pungent flavor enhances the eggs and masks the cannabis. Plus, that distinctive briny zip provides a nice contrast to the velvety egg yolks. Kalamata olives are a great choice, too.

DOSAGE WHEN MADE WITH 60% THC KIEF: ABOUT 35 MG THC PER SERVING

3 hard-boiled eggs, peeled
¼ cup finely chopped pimiento-stuffed green olives
2 tablespoons minced celery
1 tablespoon mayonnaise
¼ gram finely crumbled decarboxylated kief
1½ teaspoons whole-grain mustard
1½ teaspoons chopped fresh dill
⅛ teaspoon cayenne pepper (optional)
Salt
Freshly ground black pepper
2 small tomatoes, sliced
1 cup fresh sprouts
2 crusty bread rolls, halved

1. Finely chop the hard-boiled eggs.

2. In a medium bowl, combine the eggs, olives, celery, mayonnaise, kief, mustard, dill, cayenne (if using), season with salt and black pepper, and mix well.

3. Place the tomato slices and sprouts on the bottom half of each roll. Divide the egg salad mixture between the rolls, placing a scoop on the top half of each sandwich, and serve.

Variation tip Make this recipe vegan by substituting 1 pound of drained, soft tofu for the eggs and useing a vegan mayonnaise.

AVOCADO TOAST WITH BACON AND TOMATO

DAIRY-FREE, NUT-FREE

SERVES 4

PREP TIME:
10 MINUTES

Avocado, tomato, and bacon are a natural, palate-pleasing combo. The saltiness of the bacon and slightly sweet acidity of the tomato complement the smooth, unctuous texture of the avocado. A little decarboxylated kief instantly medicates this trendy breakfast dish.

DOSAGE WHEN MADE WITH 60% THC KIEF: ABOUT 35 MG THC PER SERVING

1 medium very ripe avocado

1 teaspoon balsamic vinegar

¼ gram finely crumbled decarboxylated kief

Salt

Freshly ground black pepper

4 thick slices sourdough bread, toasted

8 thin slices ripe tomato

8 slices cooked bacon

1. In a small bowl, mash the avocado together with the balsamic vinegar, kief, season with salt and pepper.

2. Spread the mashed avocado onto the toast slices.

3. Top each toast with 2 tomato slices and 2 bacon slices, and serve.

Variation tip Add a fried, sunny-side-up egg to the top of this toast for an even heartier breakfast.

MANGO SMOOTHIE
VEGETARIAN, GLUTEN-FREE, NUT-FREE

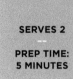

Tropical mangos and banana combine for a sunny, healthy way to start the day. Using frozen fruit gives the smoothie a thick, frosty texture without diluting the flavor with ice.

DOSAGE WHEN MADE WITH CANNABIS TINCTURE (PAGE 42): ABOUT 30 MG THC PER SERVING

1 cup frozen mango pieces
½ frozen banana
1 cup plain whole milk yogurt
½ cup milk
4 teaspoons Cannabis Tincture
   (page 42)

Place the mango, banana, yogurt, milk, and Cannabis Tincture in a blender or food processor and purée until smooth. If the smoothie is too thick, add additional milk until the desired texture is achieved.

Variation tip Turn this into India's version of a smoothie, known as a *lassi*: Simply omit the banana, substitute buttermilk for the milk, and add ½ teaspoon of ground cardamom.

HOT CAFÉ MOCHA
VEGETARIAN, GLUTEN-FREE, NUT-FREE

Chocolaty, hot café mocha is so easy to make, you'll never go to a coffeehouse again. Well, you might, but knowing you can make this at home—and medicated to boot—means fewer trips to the café and extra change in your wallet.

DOSAGE WHEN MADE WITH CANNABIS MILK OR CREAM (PAGE 39): ABOUT 40 MG THC PER SERVING

¾ **cup whole milk**

1½ **teaspoons Cannabis Milk, Cream, or Half-and-Half (page 39)**

2 **tablespoons chocolate syrup, plus additional for garnish (optional)**

¾ **cup strongly brewed hot coffee or espresso**

Whipped cream, for garnish (optional)

1. In a small saucepan, heat the milk and Cannabis Milk over low heat, watching carefully to keep the milk from reaching a boil.

2. Add the hot milk and chocolate syrup to a large coffee mug and stir until well combined. Add the coffee and stir to combine.

3. Garnish with whipped cream (if using) and additional chocolate syrup (if using).

Variation tip To make this an iced café mocha, follow the recipe through step 2, then chill the beverage. Serve over ice. For an iced blended mocha, blend the chilled mixture with 3 to 4 ice cubes until smooth. Serve immediately.

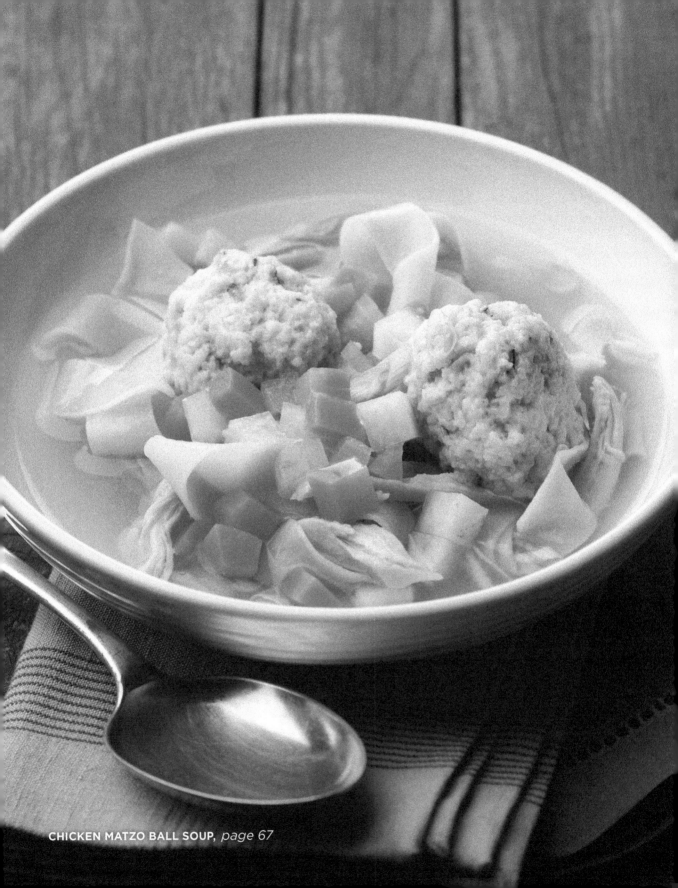

CHICKEN MATZO BALL SOUP, *page 67*

CHAPTER 6
SOUPS & SALADS

GANJA GAZPACHO
VEGAN, GLUTEN-FREE, DAIRY-FREE, NUT-FREE

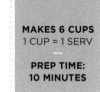

MAKES 6 CUPS
1 CUP = 1 SERV

PREP TIME:
10 MINUTES

This healthy, chilled, Spanish vegetable soup comes together quickly if you use your food processor. For the best flavor, make it in summer when garden-grown tomatoes are at their peak. It's heaven in a bowl.

DOSAGE WHEN MADE WITH CANNABIS OIL (PAGE 38): ABOUT 25 MG THC PER SERVING

5 medium ripe tomatoes

1 medium cucumber, peeled
    and seeded

1 medium yellow, orange, or red
    bell pepper

1 (12-ounce) can tomato juice

¼ cup red wine vinegar

1 or 2 jalapeño peppers, cored,
    seeded, and minced (optional)

2 tablespoons minced fresh Italian
    parsley or cilantro

2 tablespoons Cannabis Olive Oil
    (page 38)

1 tablespoon extra-virgin olive oil

1 teaspoon minced garlic

Salt

Freshly ground black pepper

1. Roughly chop (or use a food processor to roughly chop) the tomatoes, cucumber, and bell pepper. Transfer to a large bowl.

2. Stir in the tomato juice, red wine vinegar, jalapeño (if using), parsley, Cannabis Oil, olive oil, and garlic.

3. Season with salt and pepper. Stir well to combine all the ingredients. Serve cold.

Make-ahead Tip Prepare this gazpacho several hours, or even a day, in advance so the flavors have time to meld together. This recipe packs well for picnics and brown-bag lunches, too.

CHICKEN MATZO BALL SOUP
DAIRY-FREE, NUT-FREE

MAKES 8 MATZO BALLS
2 MATZO BALLS = 1 SERV

PREP TIME: 5 MINUTES,
PLUS 30 MINUTES
TO CHILL

COOK TIME: 30 MINUTES

While the garlic powder may not be traditional, it does enhance the flavor and hide some of the "green" taste, but feel free to leave it out. This soup is comfort at the highest level. When you come down with a cold, it will be your go-to meal for cozy healing.

DOSAGE WHEN MADE WITH CANNABIS OIL (PAGE 38): ABOUT 40 MG THC PER SERVING

4 eggs

¼ cup water or seltzer water

2 tablespoons Cannabis Oil (page 38)

2 tablespoons vegetable oil or schmaltz (chicken fat)

2 teaspoons garlic powder (optional)

1 teaspoon dried parsley (optional)

1 teaspoon salt

½ teaspoon freshly ground black pepper

1⅛ cups matzo meal

4 cups strong chicken stock

1 large parsnip, peeled and diced

1 large carrot, peeled and sliced into ¼-inch rounds

1 celery rib, chopped into ¼-inch pieces

1. In a medium bowl, beat the eggs, water, Cannabis Oil, and vegetable oil with a fork until well combined. Mix in the garlic powder (if using), parsley (if using), salt, and pepper. Mix in the matzo meal until thoroughly combined. Cover with plastic wrap and refrigerate for 20 to 30 minutes.

2. While waiting, bring a medium pot of salted water to a boil.

3. Pour the stock into a large pot and add the parsnip, carrot, and celery. Bring to a boil, then reduce the heat and simmer until the vegetables soften, about 10 minutes.

4. Moisten your hands with cold water and form the chilled matzo mixture into 8 balls. Drop them into the salted boiling water. Lower the heat to a simmer, cover the pot, and cook for 30 minutes. Do not open the lid.

5. Place 2 matzo balls in each bowl, and fill each with the soup and vegetables. Serve immediately.

Cooking tip A Jewish bubby (who happened to be a fabulous cook) once told me the secret to fluffy matzo balls is to *never* open the lid during cooking!

FRENCH ONION SOUP AU GRATIN

NUT-FREE

SERVES 4

—

PREP TIME:
15 MINUTES

—

COOK TIME:
1 HOUR,
10 MINUTES

For the best, most intensely flavored onion soup, take your time and sauté the onions until they are a deep brown color. In addition to making the broth richer and a little darker, caramelizing the onions brings out their natural sweetness.

DOSAGE WHEN MADE WITH 60% THC KIEF: ABOUT 35 MG PER SERVING

2 tablespoons unsalted butter

1 tablespoon extra-virgin olive oil

1 large sweet onion, such as Maui or Vidalia, thinly sliced

2 large shallots, thinly sliced

2 large leeks, white and pale green parts only, thinly sliced

1 tablespoon minced garlic

½ cup dry sherry

6 cups beef stock

1 teaspoon Worcestershire sauce

1 bay leaf

1 gram finely crumbled decarboxylated kief or hash

1 teaspoon balsamic vinegar

Salt

Freshly ground black pepper

4 slices French baguette, preferably 1 day old

1⅓ cups shredded Gruyère or Swiss cheese, divided

1. Heat the butter and olive oil in a large pot over medium heat. Add the onion, shallots, and leeks, and sauté for about 10 minutes, or until they start to brown.

2. Reduce the heat to low and continue to cook the onions until they are a deep brown, about 20 minutes, stirring every 5 minutes or so to scrape the brown bits from the bottom of the pan.

3. Add the garlic and sauté for another 2 minutes.

4. Increase the heat to medium-high and deglaze the pot with the sherry, scraping up all the brown bits from the bottom of the pot. Continue cooking until most of the sherry is gone, 2 to 3 minutes. Add the stock, Worcestershire sauce, and bay leaf. Bring to a boil, reduce the heat to low, and simmer for about 30 minutes.

5. Preheat the broiler.

6. Remove the bay leaf from the soup. Stir in the kief until it dissolves. Stir in the balsamic vinegar. Season with salt and pepper.

7. Remove the pot from the heat and divide the soup among 4 ovenproof bowls. Arrange the bowls on a baking sheet. Sprinkle ⅔ cup of cheese over the soup in the bowls. Add a baguette slice to each bowl and top it with the remaining ⅔ cup of cheese.

8. Place the baking sheet of bowls under the broiler until the cheese is melted and lightly browned, 3 to 4 minutes. Serve immediately.

Make-ahead tip Make a double batch of this soup to freeze and bake later. Cool the soup completely, then chill it before assembling as in step 7. Cover the freezer-to-oven-safe bowls with foil and freeze. Bake the frozen soup at 375°F until it is hot and the cheese is melted and browned, about 45 minutes.

CREAM OF BUTTERNUT SQUASH SOUP

GLUTEN-FREE, NUT-FREE

SERVES 4

PREP TIME:
15 MINUTES

COOK TIME:
55 MINUTES

Here's a sophisticated soup with a sweet, slightly spicy flavor, making it a perfect starter for a festive fall or winter holiday meal. Butternut squash is such a versatile food that brings warmth to any dish, whether puréed into soup or roasted with fresh sage.

DOSAGE WHEN MADE WITH CANNABIS CREAM (PAGE 39): ABOUT 25 MG THC PER SERVING

½ **large butternut squash**

1½ **teaspoons unsalted butter**

1½ **teaspoons extra-virgin olive oil**

2 **large shallots, peeled and diced**

½ **teaspoon minced garlic**

⅓ **cup freshly squeezed orange juice**

2½ **cups chicken or vegetable stock**

1 **teaspoon curry powder**

⅛ **teaspoon cayenne pepper (optional)**

Salt

Freshly ground black pepper

2 **tablespoons Cannabis Cream or Half-and-Half (page 39)**

2 **tablespoons cream or half-and-half**

1. Use a spoon to scoop out the seeds and a vegetable peeler to peel off and discard the outer layer of the squash. Cut the squash into 1-inch chunks.

2. In a large stockpot, heat the butter and olive oil over medium-high heat. Add the shallots and garlic and sauté for 1 minute. Add the cubed squash and cook, stirring frequently, for 3 minutes.

3. Add the orange juice, stir, and cook for another 2 minutes.

4. Stir in the stock, curry powder, and cayenne (if using). Season with salt and pepper.

5. Bring to a boil, then reduce the heat to low, cover, and simmer, stirring occasionally, for about 45 minutes, or until the squash is very tender.

6. Remove the pot from the heat and use an immersion blender to purée the soup. Alternatively, transfer the soup to a blender or food processor to purée, working in batches if needed.

7. Add the Cannabis Cream and cream or half-and-half and purée until combined. Serve immediately.

Variation tip Substitute cooked mashed pumpkin or other varieties of winter squash for the butternut squash.

FRUIT SALAD WITH YOGURT DRESSING

VEGETARIAN, GLUTEN-FREE, NUT-FREE

Colorful fruit salad topped with creamy orange yogurt dressing is great for breakfast and even makes a healthy dessert substitute at other times of day. The beauty of it is you can add whatever mix of seasonal fruit you have on hand.

DOSAGE WHEN MADE WITH CANNABIS HONEY (PAGE 40): ABOUT 20 MG THC PER SERVING

½ cup plain whole milk yogurt

⅛ teaspoon ground cardamom (optional)

2 tablespoons frozen orange juice concentrate

1 tablespoon Cannabis Honey or Agave Sweetener (page 40)

1 tablespoon honey or agave sweetener (optional)

¼ teaspoon vanilla extract

2½ cups chopped fresh fruit, such as berries, cantaloupe, honeydew, watermelon, bananas, peaches, grapes, or a mix of your choice

1. Place the yogurt in a medium bowl and sprinkle with the cardamom (if using). Add the orange juice concentrate, Cannabis Honey, honey or agave (if using), and vanilla extract. Mix until smooth. Refrigerate while you prepare the fruit.

2. Cut the fruit and divide it between 2 bowls. Drizzle the yogurt dressing over the top. Serve immediately.

Serving tip For an impressive presentation, cut a cantaloupe or honeydew melon in half and remove the seeds. Hollow out the center to form a bowl, leaving a thin shell. Use the melon you remove to make the fruit mixture. Fill the melon "bowls" with fruit salad, top with yogurt dressing, and serve.

MIDDLE EASTERN TABOULI
VEGAN, DAIRY-FREE, NUT-FREE

SERVES 4

—

PREP TIME: 20 MINUTES, PLUS 15 MINUTES STANDING TIME

—

COOK TIME: 3 MINUTES

Hearty, whole-grain bulgur wheat mixes with herbs and veggies in this classic Middle Eastern salad. Bulgur is a great option for vegetarians and vegans, or for a Meatless Monday meal, as it's high in protein and dietary fiber so it will leave you sated.

DOSAGE WHEN MADE WITH CANNABIS OIL (PAGE 38): ABOUT 20 MG THC PER SERVING

1⅓ cups boiling water

¾ cup dry bulgur wheat

1½ teaspoons salt

1½ cups diced, seeded ripe tomatoes

¾ cup minced scallions

¾ cup finely chopped Italian parsley

¼ cup finely chopped fresh mint

5 tablespoons freshly squeezed lemon juice

3 tablespoons extra-virgin olive oil

1 tablespoon Cannabis Olive Oil (page 38)

2 teaspoons minced garlic

Freshly ground black pepper

1. Combine the boiling water, bulgur, and salt in a large bowl. Cover and let stand for 15 minutes or until the water is absorbed and the bulgur has softened.

2. Stir in the tomatoes, scallions, parsley, mint, lemon juice, olive oil, Cannabis Oil, and garlic and mix until the ingredients are evenly combined. Season with the additional salt and pepper.

3. Chill until ready to serve. This salad is best when made several hours ahead of time. Leftovers will keep for up to 4 days in an airtight container in the refrigerator.

Make-ahead tip This nutritious salad travels well, so don't forget about this recipe when it comes time to pack a brown-bag lunch or picnic.

WEDGE SALAD WITH BLUE CHEESE DRESSING

GLUTEN-FREE, NUT-FREE

SERVES 4

—

PREP TIME:
15 MINUTES

A wedge salad feels very 1970s to many people, but it likely originated in the 1920s as iceberg lettuce became popular. Pair this classic retro salad with a bowl of soup and some fresh bread to create a complete meal.

DOSAGE WHEN MADE WITH MARIJUANA MAYONNAISE (PAGE 44): ABOUT 20 MG THC PER SERVING

6 tablespoons sour cream

1 tablespoon Marijuana Mayonnaise (page 44)

1 tablespoon freshly squeezed lemon juice

4 ounces crumbled blue cheese

2 tablespoons finely chopped chives

½ teaspoon freshly ground black pepper

¼ teaspoon salt

1 head iceberg lettuce

4 slices bacon, cooked and crumbled

2 large tomatoes, seeded and diced

2 medium avocados, peeled and diced

1. Prepare the dressing by whisking together the sour cream, Marijuana Mayonnaise, and lemon juice in a small bowl until well mixed. Stir in the blue cheese, chives, pepper, and salt.

2. Cut the lettuce into quarters. Place one quarter on each of 4 salad plates. Drizzle the dressing over the lettuce wedges and sprinkle the crumbled bacon, tomatoes, and avocado on top and around the plate. Serve immediately.

Ingredient Tip One of the secrets to a great salad is to ensure the greens are completely dry, otherwise your dressing gets diluted and you end up with a watery mess on the plate. Use a clean kitchen towel or paper towels to dry the lettuce wedges before assembling this salad.

CAESAR SALAD
NUT-FREE

SERVES 4
--
PREP TIME:
15 MINUTES

Did you know that Caesar salad is not Italian? It was invented in Tijuana, Mexico, back in 1924 at a restaurant looking to attract Americans avoiding Prohibition. Given this auspicious start, it's only fitting that you can now make a cannabis-dosed version.

DOSAGE WHEN MADE WITH CANNABIS OIL (PAGE 38): ABOUT 20 MG THC PER SERVING

FOR THE DRESSING

- **4 oil-packed anchovy fillets**
- **1 egg yolk**
- **1 tablespoon freshly squeezed lemon juice**
- **1½ teaspoons Worcestershire sauce**
- **¾ teaspoon Dijon mustard**
- **½ teaspoon minced garlic**
- **¼ cup extra-virgin olive oil**
- **1 tablespoon Cannabis Olive Oil (page 38)**
- **Salt**
- **Freshly ground black pepper**

FOR THE SALAD

- **24 romaine lettuce leaves**
- **¾ cup croutons**
- **¼ cup shaved Parmesan cheese**

TO MAKE THE DRESSING

Add the anchovy fillets, egg yolk, lemon juice, Worcestershire sauce, mustard, and garlic to a blender or food processor and process until smooth. With the machine running, drizzle in the olive oil and Cannabis Oil in a slow, steady stream and process until the mixture is emulsified. Season with salt and pepper.

TO MAKE THE SALAD

Assemble the salad by arranging the romaine leaves on plates. Drizzle with the dressing, then sprinkle with the croutons and shaved Parmesan cheese. Serve immediately.

Serving tip Turn this side dish salad into a complete meal by adding grilled chicken breast, shrimp, or scallops.

CLASSIC COLESLAW
VEGETARIAN, GLUTEN-FREE, DAIRY-FREE, NUT-FREE

Some foods are classics for a reason, like this crunchy, sweet, and creamy coleslaw. To give it a south-of-the-border spicy flair, omit the mustard and add part or all (depending on how spicy you want it) of a finely chopped chipotle chile pepper in adobo sauce. It gives the coleslaw a nice smoky flavor and a kick of heat.

DOSAGE WHEN MADE WITH MARIJUANA MAYONNAISE (PAGE 44): ABOUT 30 MG THC PER SERVING

½ **cup Marijuana Mayonnaise (page 44)**
¼ **cup mayonnaise**
1 tablespoon Dijon mustard
1 tablespoon freshly squeezed lemon juice
1 teaspoon sugar
Salt
Freshly ground black pepper
1 (1-pound) bag shredded coleslaw mix containing red and green cabbage and carrots

In a large bowl, whisk together the Marijuana Mayonnaise, mayonnaise, mustard, lemon juice, and sugar. Season with salt and pepper. Add the coleslaw mix and toss until well coated. Chill until ready to serve.

Variation Tip Adding 1 cup of golden raisins or sweetened dried cranberries to this slaw provides a tasty element of surprise.

CHINESE CHICKEN SALAD
DAIRY-FREE

Sweet and savory come together in this fabulous main-dish salad. Plus, it's a great way to use up leftover cooked chicken. While the dressing is easy to make, the complex flavors of ginger, soy sauce, and sesame will dance on your tongue.

DOSAGE WHEN MADE WITH CANNABIS OIL (PAGE 38): ABOUT 20 MG THC PER SERVING

FOR THE DRESSING
⅛ **cup rice vinegar**
1 **tablespoon toasted sesame seeds**
2 **teaspoons freshly grated ginger**
2 **teaspoons soy sauce**
2 **teaspoons brown sugar**
1 **teaspoon sesame oil**
⅛ **teaspoon minced garlic**
Salt
½ **teaspoon freshly ground black pepper**
1 **tablespoon neutral Cannabis Oil (page 38)**
1 **tablespoon vegetable or canola oil**

FOR THE SALAD
6 **cups shredded napa cabbage**
2 **cups shredded red cabbage**
1 **cup shredded carrots**
½ **cup chopped scallions**
1 **(11-ounce) can mandarin oranges, drained**
2 **cups chopped or shredded cooked chicken**
¼ **cup sliced almonds, toasted**

TO MAKE THE DRESSING
Stir together the rice vinegar, sesame seeds, ginger, soy sauce, brown sugar, sesame oil, garlic, season with salt, and add pepper. Vigorously whisk in the Cannabis Oil and vegetable oil in a slow, steady stream to mix and emulsify the dressing. Alternatively, combine these ingredients in a blender or food processor.

TO MAKE THE SALAD
1. In a large bowl, combine the napa cabbage, red cabbage, carrots, scallions, mandarin oranges, and cooked chicken. Drizzle with the dressing, then toss together to coat.

2. Divide the salad among 4 plates, and garnish each with the toasted almond slices. Serve immediately.

Cooking tip To toast the almonds, heat a small skillet over medium-high heat. Add the sliced almonds to the dry skillet and cook, stirring frequently, until light brown, about 5 minutes.

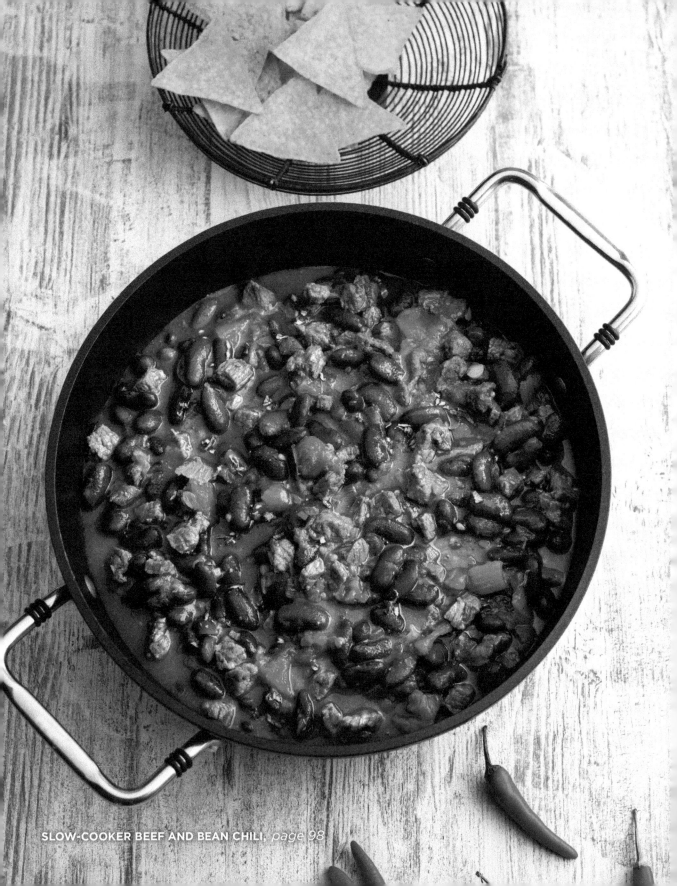

SLOW-COOKER BEEF AND BEAN CHILI, *page 98*

CHAPTER 7
MAIN MEALS

CHEESY FETTUCCINE ALFREDO
VEGETARIAN, NUT-FREE

Rich, creamy, and cheesy fettuccine Alfredo makes the ultimate indulgent pasta entrée. For some variety and crunch, try adding a little healthy color to the plate by mixing in some steamed veggies like broccoli, carrots, or zucchini.

DOSAGE WHEN MADE WITH CANNABIS BUTTER (PAGE 37): ABOUT 25 MG THC PER SERVING

1½ pounds fresh or dried fettuccine

½ cup plus 2 tablespoons unsalted butter

2 tablespoons Cannabis Butter (page 37)

1 tablespoon minced garlic

2 cups half-and-half or heavy (whipping) cream

Salt

1 teaspoon freshly ground black or white pepper

¾ cup (3 ounces) grated Parmesan cheese

1 cup (4 ounces) shredded whole milk mozzarella cheese

1. Cook the fettuccine according to the package directions. Drain and set aside.

2. In a large saucepan, melt the butter and Cannabis Butter over medium-low heat. Add the garlic and cook, stirring often, for 30 seconds. Add the half-and-half, season with salt, and add the pepper. Bring to a simmer, stirring frequently and watching carefully to prevent the pot from boiling over, which can happen quickly.

3. Stir in the Parmesan and cook, stirring constantly, for 5 minutes. Stir in the mozzarella and continue to cook until the cheese melts, about 5 minutes. Remove the pan from the heat and whisk or use an immersion blender to smooth the sauce. Pour over the hot cooked pasta and serve.

Serving tip This recipe yields about 3 cups of sauce that has plenty of uses beyond topping pasta. Try pairing it with simple grilled or steamed chicken, fish, or vegetables.

BAKED JALAPEÑO MAC AND CHEESE

VEGETARIAN, NUT-FREE

SERVES 8

PREP TIME:
15 MINUTES

COOK TIME:
45 MINUTES

The ultimate comfort food, this creamy mac and cheese with a crunchy baked crust has just the right hint of spice. Of course, you can always skip the jalapeño, but the slight kick of heat offers an unexpected and delightful twist on a classic preparation.

DOSAGE WHEN MADE WITH CANNABIS BUTTER (PAGE 37): ABOUT 20 MG THC PER SERVING

FOR THE MACARONI

Salt

1 pound elbow macaroni

2 tablespoons Cannabis Butter (page 37)

2 tablespoons unsalted butter

3 large jalapeños, 2 finely chopped and 1 thinly sliced, divided

2½ cups half-and-half

8 ounces cream cheese

4 ounces (about 1½ cups) shredded sharp Cheddar cheese

4 ounces (about 1½ cups) shredded pepper Jack cheese

⅛ to ¼ teaspoon cayenne pepper

Freshly ground black pepper

FOR THE TOPPING

¼ cup unsalted butter, melted

1 cup panko bread crumbs

TO MAKE THE MACARONI

1. Set an oven rack in the upper third of the oven and preheat to 375°F.

2. Bring a large pot of salted water to a boil. Add the macaroni and cook until al dente, about 5 minutes. Strain, reserving 1¾ cups of the pasta water. Set the strained pasta and reserved water aside.

3. In the same pot, melt the Cannabis Butter and butter over medium heat. Add the chopped jalapeños and cook, stirring often, until softened, about 5 minutes. Transfer to a small bowl and set aside.

4. Add the half-and-half to the pot. Cook over medium heat until it just comes to a simmer. Reduce the heat to low and continue simmering until the half-and-half is reduced to 1½ cups, about 10 minutes.

5. Add the cream cheese and stir until it is melted into the cream.

6. Whisk in the Cheddar and pepper Jack cheeses until melted and the sauce is smooth.

Continued

7. Add the macaroni and reserved pasta water and stir until well combined. Season with the cayenne, salt, and black pepper.

8. Transfer to a 13-by-9-inch baking dish.

TO MAKE THE TOPPING

1. Mix the melted butter with the panko crumbs.

2. Spread an even, thin layer of the topping over the macaroni and cheese. Arrange the jalapeño slices on top of the bread crumbs. Bake until the mac and cheese is bubbly and the topping is lightly browned, about 20 minutes.

Cooking tip Don't worry if things look soupy after step 7. Looks can be deceiving at this stage and the macaroni will absorb the excess sauce as it bakes.

SHRIMP CREOLE
NUT-FREE

SERVES 4
--
PREP TIME:
10 MINUTES
--
COOK TIME:
35 MINUTES

Sweet shrimp swim in a spicy tomato sauce in this classic Creole dish. The flavors of the other ingredients are subtle enough to complement the shrimp rather than overpower it. Serve over white or brown rice to soak up every bit of sauce.

DOSAGE WHEN MADE WITH CANNABIS OIL (PAGE 38): ABOUT 20 MG THC PER SERVING

1 tablespoon unsalted butter

1 tablespoon extra-virgin olive oil

2 tablespoons all-purpose flour

½ small onion, diced

½ small green bell pepper, cored and diced

1 large celery rib, finely diced

2 teaspoons minced garlic

1 (15-ounce) can crushed tomatoes

1 cup chicken or vegetable stock

2 tablespoons chopped fresh Italian parsley or 2 teaspoons dried parsley

1 tablespoon Cannabis Oil (page 38)

1 bay leaf

⅛ teaspoon cayenne pepper

Salt

1 pound medium shrimp, peeled

Cooked rice

1. In a large skillet, melt the butter with the olive oil over medium heat. Whisk in the flour and cook, whisking constantly, until a light brown roux forms, 3 to 4 minutes.

2. Add the onion, bell pepper, and celery to the pan and stir with a wooden spoon to combine. Cook, stirring constantly, until the vegetables are softened, about 4 minutes.

3. Stir in the garlic and cook for 1 minute more.

4. Stir in the tomatoes and their juices, stock, parsley, Cannabis Oil, bay leaf, cayenne, and salt. Increase the heat and bring the mixture to a boil. Then reduce the heat and simmer for about 15 minutes.

5. Add the shrimp, stirring to combine, and cook just until the shrimp are no longer translucent, 4 to 5 minutes. Carefully remove the bay leaf, and serve over the cooked rice.

Cooking tip One of the first and most important lessons instilled in any competent Creole chef is to never leave a roux while it's on the stove. The cooking combination of equal parts flour and fat can turn into a burned mess in seconds. Stir constantly.

STIR-FRIED SCALLOPS AND ASPARAGUS

GLUTEN-FREE, NUT-FREE

SERVES 4

—

PREP TIME:
15 MINUTES

COOK TIME:
12 MINUTES

This elegant stir-fry dinner comes together in a flash. The velvety, creamy texture of the scallops perfectly contrasts with the crisp crunch of the asparagus. Serve over rice or your favorite Asian-style noodles.

DOSAGE WHEN MADE WITH CANNABIS BUTTER (PAGE 37): ABOUT 20 MG THC PER SERVING

⅓ **cup chicken or vegetable stock**

2 **tablespoons minced fresh ginger**

2 **tablespoons rice vinegar**

2 **tablespoons oyster sauce**

1 **tablespoon sesame oil**

2 **teaspoons cornstarch**

1 **teaspoon sugar**

½ **teaspoon minced garlic**

½ **teaspoon freshly ground black pepper**

2 **tablespoons unsalted butter, melted**

1 **tablespoon Cannabis Butter (page 37), melted**

4 **teaspoons vegetable or canola oil, divided**

1 **pound fresh small scallops**

2 **cups fresh trimmed asparagus pieces (each stalk cut into 4 to 5 pieces)**

2 **cups sliced white, cremini, or shiitake mushrooms**

4 **scallions, minced**

1. Whisk together the stock, ginger, rice vinegar, oyster sauce, sesame oil, cornstarch, sugar, garlic, and pepper until well combined. Whisk in the melted butter and Cannabis Butter until well combined and the mixture is emulsified. Alternatively, prepare this sauce in a small food processor. Set aside.

2. Heat a wok over high heat. Add 2 teaspoons of vegetable oil and swirl to coat the wok. Add the scallops and stir-fry just until cooked, 4 to 5 minutes. Transfer the scallops to a bowl and set aside.

3. Add the remaining 2 teaspoons of vegetable oil to the wok and swirl to coat. Add the asparagus, mushrooms, and scallions and stir-fry until crisp-tender, about 6 minutes.

4. Return the scallops to the wok and stir to combine with the vegetables. Stir the sauce and pour it into the wok. Cook, stirring constantly, for about 1 minute or until the sauce heats through, thickens, and evenly coats the food. Serve immediately over rice or noodles.

Ingredient Tip Oyster sauce, a staple of Chinese cuisine, is a thick, dark brown condiment made from ground dried oysters. Available at Asian food markets or well-stocked grocery stores, oyster sauce will keep indefinitely in your refrigerator.

GRILLED FISH TACOS WITH GREEN CHILE SALSA

GLUTEN-FREE, NUT-FREE

SERVES 2

--

PREP TIME:
15 MINUTES

--

COOK TIME:
12 MINUTES

These grilled fish tacos are lighter, healthier, and far less messy to make than their fried counterparts. The medicated, mild green chile salsa ties everything together. Be sure to use a firm-fleshed fish, otherwise it becomes mushy.

DOSAGE WHEN MADE WITH CANNABIS OIL (PAGE 38): ABOUT 20 MG THC PER SERVING

FOR THE SALSA

1 large mild green chile,
 preferably Anaheim
1 small jalapeño
1 medium tomatillo, husk
 removed, halved
½ small yellow onion
⅓ cup cilantro
1½ teaspoons Cannabis Oil (page 38)
½ teaspoon minced garlic
Juice of 1 lime
Salt
Freshly ground black pepper

FOR THE TACOS

1 pound halibut, mahimahi, or other
 firm-fleshed fish
1 teaspoon vegetable oil
Salt
Freshly ground black pepper
4 large corn tortillas
1 cup shredded cabbage
1 medium avocado, sliced
⅓ cup crumbled queso fresco

TO MAKE THE SALSA

1. Preheat the grill to medium-high heat.

2. Grill the green chile, jalapeño, tomatillo, and onion, turning with tongs until each side is lightly charred.

3. Place the hot chiles and jalapeño in a paper bag and close it. Let the bag sit for 5 minutes, then run the peppers under water to easily peel away the outer skin. Remove the stems and seeds.

4. Transfer the chiles, onion, and tomatillo to a food processor or blender along with the cilantro, Cannabis Oil, garlic, and lime juice. Process on high until smooth. Season with salt and pepper and set aside.

TO MAKE THE TACOS

1. Brush the fish with the vegetable oil and season with the salt and pepper on both sides. Grill over a medium-hot fire for 2 to 3 minutes per side, or until the fish is done to your liking or flakes easily with a fork.

2. Heat the tortillas for about 15 seconds per side over the grill. Place a layer of shredded cabbage on each tortilla, top with the grilled fish, salsa, sliced avocado, and crumbled cheese. Serve immediately.

Ingredient tip Contrary to popular belief, a chile's heat is *not* held in its seeds, but rather the white inner membrane. If you want less heat and more chile flavor, take care to remove this part. Always wash your hands well after preparing chiles.

SESAME HONEY LIME CHICKEN
DAIRY-FREE, NUT-FREE

You can grill or bake the chicken for this recipe. I like to serve it with rice to soak up every drop of the tangy-sweet cannabis-infused glaze. Quinoa or orzo will do the trick, too. So does just licking the plate!

DOSAGE WHEN MADE WITH CANNABIS HONEY (PAGE 40): ABOUT 20 MG THC PER SERVING

1 chicken, cut into 8 pieces
Salt
Freshly ground black pepper
¼ cup light soy sauce
6 tablespoons honey
2 tablespoons Cannabis Honey (page 40)
2 tablespoons freshly squeezed lime juice
1 teaspoon sriracha hot sauce
1 teaspoon grated fresh ginger
½ teaspoon sesame oil
2 teaspoons toasted sesame seeds
Chopped scallions, for garnish (optional)
3 cups cooked rice

1. Preheat a grill to medium-hot or the oven to 375°F.

2. Season the chicken pieces with the salt and pepper. Cook on the grill fire, turning once, until cooked through, or in the oven, about 40 minutes.

3. While the chicken is cooking, prepare the glaze. In a small saucepan, combine the soy sauce, honey, Cannabis Honey, lime juice, sriracha, ginger, and sesame oil. Heat over medium-low heat, stirring constantly, until the mixture starts to bubble. Watch carefully because it can bubble over in seconds. Reduce the heat to low and continue to cook, stirring constantly, until the glaze is slightly thickened, about 3 minutes.

4. Place the cooked chicken in a large bowl and toss with the glaze to coat. Garnish with the sesame seeds and scallions (if using) and serve over the rice.

Substitution tip In a huge hurry? Use restaurant or store-bought rotisserie, grilled, or even fried chicken, then just toss with the medicated glaze.

CHICKEN CURRY
GLUTEN-FREE, NUT-FREE

SERVES 4

—

PREP TIME:
15 MINUTES

—

COOK TIME:
23 MINUTES

Indian curry-spiced yogurt sauce envelops tender pieces of white-meat chicken in this easy-to-prepare recipe. Serve over fragrant jasmine or basmati rice. To make a Thai curry, use coconut milk in place of the yogurt.

DOSAGE WHEN MADE WITH CANNABIS OIL (PAGE 38): ABOUT 20 MG THC PER SERVING

2 tablespoons vegetable or extra-virgin olive oil

1½ pounds boneless, skinless chicken breasts, cut into 1-inch cubes

1 large onion, diced

1 jalapeño pepper, cored, seeded and minced

1 tablespoon Cannabis Oil (page 38)

1 tablespoon curry powder

2 teaspoons grated fresh ginger

1½ teaspoons minced garlic

½ teaspoon turmeric

½ cup whole milk plain yogurt

½ cup chicken stock

¼ cup minced cilantro

Salt

Freshly ground black pepper

3 cups cooked jasmine or basmati rice

1. In a large skillet, heat the vegetable oil over medium-high heat. Add the chicken, onion, and jalapeño and cook, stirring frequently with a wooden spoon, until the chicken begins to brown and the onion is softened and translucent, about 5 minutes.

2. Stir in the Cannabis Oil, curry powder, ginger, garlic, and turmeric and mix until well combined. Reduce the heat to medium-low. Add the yogurt and cook, stirring constantly, until thickened, about 3 minutes.

3. Stir in the chicken stock and cilantro. Season with salt and pepper.

4. Reduce the heat to low and cover the skillet. Simmer, stirring occasionally, for about 15 minutes or until the chicken is cooked through. Serve over the cooked rice.

Storage tip This dish freezes well, so you can enjoy it another day when you need a quick meal. In an airtight freezer-safe container, top the cooled cooked rice with cooled curry and freeze. When ready to eat, microwave the frozen curry on high, stopping to stir every minute or so, until heated through.

BARBECUE CHICKEN
GLUTEN-FREE, DAIRY-FREE, NUT-FREE

SERVES 4

PREP TIME:
10 MINUTES

COOK TIME:
40 MINUTES

If you like your barbecue sauce spicy, add a dash or two of cayenne pepper. If not, leave it out for a thick, sweet, slightly vinegary barbecue sauce. Use this versatile sauce to medicate all kinds of other grilled meats.

DOSAGE WHEN MADE WITH CANNABIS OIL (PAGE 38): ABOUT 20 MG THC PER SERVING

½ cup diced yellow or white onion
1 tablespoon water
2 teaspoons extra-virgin olive oil
½ cup ketchup
⅛ cup packed brown sugar
1 tablespoon apple cider vinegar
1 tablespoon Cannabis Oil (page 38)
2 teaspoons Worcestershire sauce
¾ teaspoon liquid smoke
½ teaspoon minced garlic
½ teaspoon oregano
½ teaspoon dry mustard powder
Cayenne pepper (optional)
Salt
Freshly ground black pepper
1 chicken, cut into 8 pieces

1. Place the onion and water in a food processor or blender and purée until smooth.

2. Heat a small saucepan over medium heat and add the olive oil. Add the onion purée and cook, stirring often, 2 to 3 minutes.

3. Add the ketchup, brown sugar, cider vinegar, Cannabis Oil, Worcestershire sauce, liquid smoke, garlic, oregano, mustard powder, and cayenne (if using) and mix until well combined. Bring the sauce to a simmer, then reduce the heat to low. Cover the pan and simmer, stirring occasionally, for 10 minutes. Season with salt and pepper.

4. Grill the chicken over medium-hot heat, turning once, until cooked through, about 40 minutes.

5. Remove the chicken from the grill and let it rest for 5 minutes. Place the cooked chicken pieces in a large bowl, pour the sauce over, and toss to coat.

Ingredient Tip Liquid smoke is a seasoning made from concentrated hickory or mesquite smoke. It imparts a distinctive smoky flavor to foods, so a little goes a long way. Find liquid smoke in most grocery stores along with the steak sauces.

CHICKEN AND SAUSAGE JAMBALAYA

GLUTEN-FREE, DAIRY-FREE, NUT-FREE

SERVES 6

PREP TIME:
10 MINUTES

COOK TIME:
45 MINUTES

I created this easy jambalaya recipe to come together fast for a satisfying, anytime dinner. Since it only uses one pot, you'll even save time on cleanup. Of the many delicious and distinctive regional cuisines in America, these Creole and Cajun flavors of Louisiana are among the most unique and influential.

DOSAGE WHEN MADE WITH CANNABIS OIL (PAGE 38): ABOUT 25 MG THC PER SERVING

- 2 teaspoons extra-virgin olive oil
- 1 pound boneless, skinless chicken breasts, cut into 1-inch pieces
- 1 pound smoked sausage, cut into 1-inch pieces
- 2 medium yellow onions, diced
- 2 large celery stalks, diced
- 1 large green bell pepper, cored, seeded, and diced
- 1¼ cups uncooked white or brown rice
- 2 tablespoons Cannabis Oil (page 38)
- 2 teaspoons minced garlic
- 4 cups chicken stock
- 2 bay leaves
- 1 teaspoon dried thyme
- 1 teaspoon dried oregano
- 1 teaspoon hot sauce, such as Tabasco
- ½ teaspoon salt
- ¼ teaspoon cayenne pepper

1. Heat the olive oil in a large pot over medium-high heat. Add the chicken and cook, stirring often, until browned, about 5 minutes.

2. Add the sausage, onions, celery, and green pepper and cook, stirring frequently, for about 10 minutes, or until the onion has started to brown.

3. Stir in the rice, Cannabis Oil, and garlic and cook, stirring constantly, for about 1 minute.

4. Stir in the chicken stock, scraping up any browned bits on the bottom of the pan.

5. Add the bay leaves, and stir in the thyme, oregano, hot sauce, salt, and cayenne. Reduce the heat to low, cover, and simmer, stirring occasionally, for 25 minutes or until most of the liquid is absorbed and the rice is tender. Carefully remove the bay leaf, and serve immediately.

Storage Tip Freeze in airtight containers for up to 4 months. When ready to eat, microwave the thawed or frozen jambalaya, stirring frequently, until heated through.

ITALIAN SUB SANDWICH
NUT-FREE

SERVES 1
—
PREP TIME:
15 MINUTES

The unmedicated version of this recipe was one of the most popular menu items at the Italian restaurant I used to own. This cannabis-enhanced creation is even better. As with a proper Italian sub, you can simultaneously taste the individual ingredients and a melding of flavors in every bite.

DOSAGE WHEN MADE WITH CANNABIS OIL (PAGE 38): ABOUT 20 MG THC PER SERVING

1 sandwich-size Italian roll
2 teaspoons balsamic vinegar
1 teaspoon Cannabis Olive Oil (page 38)
1 teaspoon extra-virgin olive oil
1½ tablespoons minced pepperoncinis
½ cup finely chopped lettuce
2 tablespoons chopped tomatoes
1½ tablespoons red onion
2 slices smoked deli ham
3 slices mortadella
4 slices Genoa salami
3 slices spicy *capocollo*
2 slices provolone cheese

1. Slice off the top third of the roll lengthwise. Remove some of the inner bread filling (creating a shallow well) and reserve for another use like bread crumbs.

2. Lightly add a sprinkling of the balsamic vinegar, Cannabis Oil, and olive oil to both cut sides of the bread.

3. Add the pepperoncinis to the well in the bottom half of the bread, followed by the lettuce, tomato, and red onion.

4. Fold the ham slices in half lengthwise and place on top of the vegetables, followed by the mortadella. Add the salami and *capocollo* and top with cheese.

5. Close the sandwich with the top half of the roll, cut, and serve.

Cooking tip This sandwich is delicious cold, but it's also great hot. Place both bread halves on a baking sheet. Divide the meats evenly among the seasoned bottom and top halves of bread. Distribute the vegetables among the two halves. Place under a preheated broiler for 3 to 4 minutes or until the meat is heated and the cheese is melty. Remove from the oven, place both bread halves together, and serve.

APPLE-STUFFED PORK CHOPS

DAIRY-FREE, NUT-FREE

SERVES 2

PREP TIME:
20 MINUTES

COOK TIME:
53 MINUTES

Need a medicated entrée for a special meal? Look no further than juicy pork chops stuffed with cornbread, tart apples, and smoky bacon. Savory and satisfying, this dish is a modern, healthier twist.

DOSAGE WHEN MADE WITH CANNABIS OIL (PAGE 38): ABOUT 20 MG THC PER SERVING

Nonstick cooking spray

1 slice bacon

½ small onion, finely diced

1 small Granny Smith apple, peeled, cored, and finely diced

1 cup dried cornbread cubes

3 tablespoons minced fresh Italian parsley or 1 tablespoon dried parsley

½ cup chicken stock

1½ teaspoons Cannabis Oil (page 38)

Salt

Freshly ground black pepper

2 (1¼-inch thick) bone-in rib or loin pork chops

1. Preheat the oven to 350°F. Spray a baking dish with nonstick cooking spray.

2. Cut the bacon into small pieces and cook them in a medium skillet over medium heat, stirring occasionally, until crisp, about 5 minutes.

3. Add the onion and cook for 2 to 3 minutes, or until softened and starting to brown.

4. Remove the skillet from the heat and stir in the apple, cornbread cubes, and parsley. Add the chicken stock and Cannabis Oil, and season with salt and pepper. Mix until well combined. The bread cubes will absorb the liquid.

5. Use a sharp knife to make a pocket in each pork chop by cutting through the meat toward the bone. Fill each pocket with the stuffing and place them in the prepared baking dish.

6. Bake, uncovered, for about 45 minutes or until the chops are browned and the meat is cooked through. Let rest for 5 minutes before serving.

Substitution tip For a nice variation, try replacing the apples in the stuffing with peeled diced peaches—especially in summer months when they are in season.

ASIAN-STYLE STEAK SALAD
DAIRY-FREE, NUT-FREE

SERVES 4

—

PREP TIME:
10 MINUTES

—

COOK TIME:
10 MINUTES

Flame-kissed grilled steak tops healthy greens and colorful veggies coated in a tangy, lime-based dressing for an Asian-inspired main course salad.

DOSAGE WHEN MADE WITH CANNABIS OIL (PAGE 38): ABOUT 20 MG THC PER SERVING

1 pound lean sirloin steak

Salt

Freshly ground black pepper

3 tablespoons vegetable or canola oil

2 tablespoons freshly squeezed lime juice

1 tablespoon Cannabis Oil (page 38)

1 tablespoon low-sodium soy sauce

1½ teaspoons fish sauce

¾ teaspoon sesame oil

½ teaspoon sriracha hot sauce (optional)

½ teaspoon sugar

½ teaspoon minced garlic

8 cups Asian salad greens blend

½ cup chopped cilantro

¼ cup chopped fresh mint

8 large radishes, sliced

1 large cucumber, peeled and sliced

1 large carrot, shredded

¼ large red onion, thinly sliced

1. Preheat the grill to medium-high heat.

2. Season the steak with salt and pepper and grill to rare or medium-rare doneness, about 5 minutes on each side. Remove the steak from the heat and let it rest while you prepare the rest of the salad.

3. Prepare the dressing by whisking together the vegetable oil, lime juice, Cannabis Oil, soy sauce, fish sauce, sesame oil, sriracha (if using), sugar, and garlic until well combined and emulsified.

4. In a large bowl, toss together the salad greens, cilantro, and mint. Add the dressing and toss to coat the greens.

5. Divide the greens among 4 large plates.

6. Slice the steak across the grain and arrange the slices on top of the greens.

7. Surround the edges of each plate with the radishes, cucumber, and carrot. Top the salad with rings of red onion and serve immediately.

Variation tip Divide the beef and veggies between 8 large iceberg or butter lettuce leaves. Wrap the lettuce leaves around the filling to make 8 rolls. Serve 2 lettuce wraps per person with dressing alongside for dipping.

GRILLED FLANK STEAK WITH CHIMICHURRI SAUCE

GLUTEN-FREE, DAIRY-FREE, NUT-FREE

SERVES 6

PREP TIME: 10 MINUTES

COOK TIME: 10 MINUTES, PLUS 5 MINUTES TO REST

This classic South American sauce of parsley, lemon, and garlic makes the perfect accompaniment to grilled meats. I like flank steak because it is flavorful and lean, but you could spoon this aromatic, pungent sauce on any of your favorite cuts of beef.

DOSAGE WHEN MADE WITH CANNABIS OIL (PAGE 38): ABOUT 25 MG THC PER SERVING

1¼ cup Italian parsley

⅔ cup extra-virgin olive oil

⅓ cup freshly squeezed lemon juice

2 tablespoons Cannabis Olive Oil (page 38)

2 tablespoons minced garlic

1 teaspoon salt, plus additional to season the steak

1 teaspoon freshly ground black pepper, plus additional to season the steak

½ teaspoon crushed red pepper

1½ pounds flank steak, at room temperature

1. Preheat the grill to medium-hot heat.

2. Combine the parsley, olive oil, lemon juice, Cannabis Oil, garlic, salt, black pepper, and crushed red pepper in a blender or food processor, and process to purée and combine ingredients. Set aside.

3. Season both sides of the steak with salt and black pepper. Grill the steak for about 5 minutes per side for medium-rare, or until it reaches the preferred doneness. Remove the steak from the heat and let it rest for 5 minutes before cutting.

4. Slice the steak against the grain and serve accompanied by chimichurri sauce.

Variation tip While it might not be traditional, chimichurri sauce is also delicious served over hot grilled pork, chicken, fish, or even tofu.

SERVES 6
½ LOAF = 1 SERV

PREP TIME:
15 MINUTES

COOK TIME:
55 MINUTES

MOTA MEATLOAF

DAIRY-FREE, NUT-FREE

Kicked up with spicy jalapeños and *mota* (the Spanish word for marijuana), then coated in a sweet-and-spicy glaze, this is not your grandma's meatloaf. The combination of homey comfort food with medicating kief will have you feeling better in no time.

DOSAGE WHEN MADE WITH 60% THC KIEF: ABOUT 25 MG THC PER SERVING

FOR THE MEATLOAF

Cooking spray

1½ pounds lean ground beef

1 pound ground pork

1½ grams decarboxylated kief

1 or 2 jalapeño peppers, cored, seeded, and minced

1 medium white or yellow onion, finely chopped

¾ cup dry bread crumbs

2 teaspoons minced garlic

1½ teaspoons salt

1½ teaspoons freshly ground black pepper

1 teaspoon dried thyme

1 teaspoon dried oregano

1 egg, lightly beaten

FOR THE GLAZE

⅓ cup ketchup

1 tablespoon Worcestershire sauce

1 teaspoon chili powder

½ teaspoon soy sauce

Hot sauce

TO MAKE THE MEATLOAF

1. Preheat the oven to 325°F. Spray a large rimmed baking sheet liberally with cooking spray.

2. Place the ground beef and pork in a large bowl. Sprinkle the kief over the meat and use clean hands to thoroughly mix the cannabis into the meat.

3. Add the jalapeño, onion, bread crumbs, garlic, salt, pepper, thyme, oregano, and egg, and continue to mix until all the ingredients are evenly combined.

4. Use a 3¾-by-6½-inch loaf pan to form a third of the meat into a loaf shape, then carefully remove it from the pan and place the loaf on the prepared baking pan. Repeat with the remaining meat for a total of 3 loaves. Bake for 15 minutes.

TO MAKE THE GLAZE

While the meatloaf bakes, prepare the glaze by mixing together the ketchup, Worcestershire sauce, chili powder, soy sauce, and hot sauce until well combined. Use a pastry brush to smooth glaze on the tops and sides of each loaf. Continue to bake the meatloaf until cooked though and browned on top, about 40 minutes more. Let rest for 10 minutes before slicing and serving.

Note. While I tested the recipe using a small (3¾-by-6½-inch) loaf pan, you can make the loaf any size you like. Just keep in mind a single-dose serving is one-sixth of the total recipe.

SLOW-COOKER BEEF AND BEAN CHILI

GLUTEN-FREE, DAIRY-FREE, NUT-FREE

SERVES 4

—

PREP TIME:
20 MINUTES

—

COOK TIME:
4 TO 6 HOURS

Using a slow cooker lets you prep this recipe early in the day and forget about it until dinnertime. Nothing beats coming home to a hot, comforting meal that's all ready to be dished up. Your taste buds will enjoy the beauty of a slow cooker, too.

DOSAGE WHEN MADE WITH CANNABIS OIL (PAGE 38): ABOUT 20 MG THC PER SERVING

- 2 ounces dried chiles, such as New Mexico, California, guajillo, pasilla, or a combination, about 6 to 8 chiles total
- 1 corn tortilla
- 1 tablespoon Cannabis Oil (page 38)
- 1 tablespoon salt
- 2 teaspoons freshly ground black pepper
- 1½ teaspoons ground cumin
- 1 teaspoon dried oregano
- ½ teaspoon cayenne pepper (optional)
- 3½ cups beef stock, divided

- 4 teaspoons extra-virgin olive oil, divided
- 3 pounds boneless beef chuck, trimmed of fat and cut into ¾-inch chunks, about 2½ pounds after trimming
- 1 medium yellow onion, diced
- 1 tablespoon minced garlic
- 1 (15-ounce) can kidney beans, drained
- ½ cup black coffee
- 2 tablespoons cider vinegar
- 1 tablespoon brown sugar

1. Place the chiles in a cast-iron skillet over medium-low heat and toast until fragrant, about 2 minutes per side. Be careful not to burn as that will turn the chiles bitter. Place the toasted chiles in a bowl, cover them with boiling water, and soak until they are soft, about 20 minutes, turning them once or twice.

2. Heat the tortilla in the dry skillet to toast it, about 1 minute on each side. Remove it from the heat. When it's cool enough to handle, tear it into pieces. Pulse the pieces into fine crumbs in a blender or food processor. Set aside.

3. Drain the chiles, then split them open to remove the stems and seeds. Place the seeded chiles in a blender or food processor with the Cannabis Oil, salt, black pepper, cumin, oregano, and cayenne (if using). Purée the mixture, then add 2 cups of beef stock, and continue to blend until you have a smooth paste. Transfer this to the slow cooker set on high.

4. Return the skillet to medium-high heat and add 2 teaspoons of olive oil. Brown the beef in two batches, turning each piece to brown all sides. Drain and add the cooked beef to the slow cooker.

5. Add the remaining 2 teaspoons of olive oil to the skillet and add the onion and garlic and cook, stirring often, until the onion just starts to brown, about 2 minutes. Transfer to the slow cooker.

6. Add the puréed tortilla, beans, remaining 1½ cups of beef stock, coffee, cider vinegar, and brown sugar to the slow cooker and stir to blend well. Cover and let cook for 4 to 6 hours or until the beef is tender.

Serving tip Let your guests "play with their food" by offering an array of garnishes and condiments along with the bowls of chili. Grated Cheddar cheese, diced raw onion, sour cream, and a selection of your favorite hot sauces make good additions.

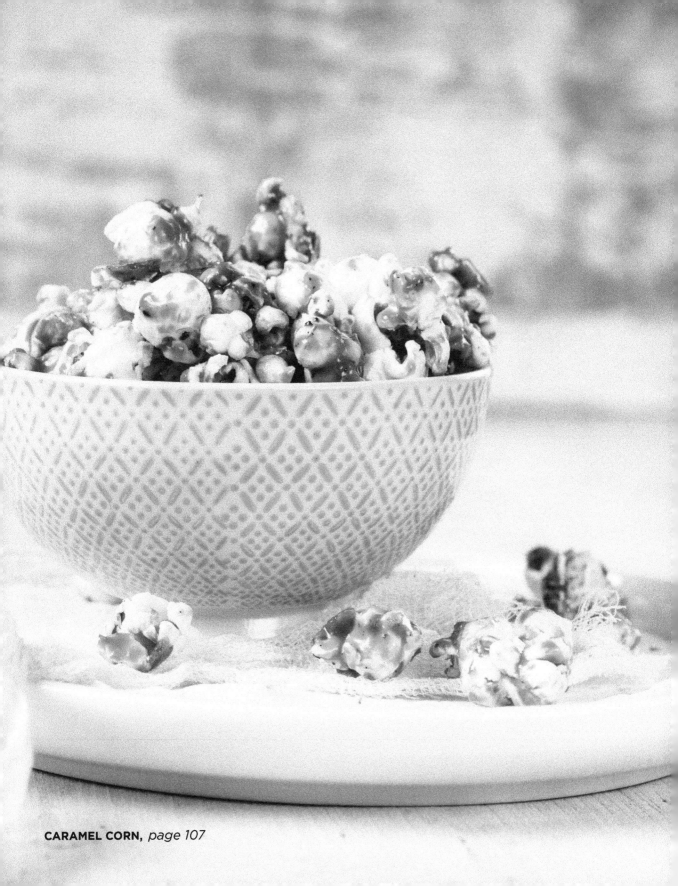

CARAMEL CORN, *page 107*

CHAPTER 8
SNACKS

HEMP HUMMUS
VEGAN, GLUTEN-FREE, DAIRY-FREE, NUT-FREE

Serve this healthy Mediterranean dip with raw vegetables or triangles of pita bread. It also makes a terrific, high-protein, vegetarian sandwich spread. Don't be confused when ingredient shopping—garbanzo beans and chickpeas are different names for the exact same legume.

DOSAGE WHEN MADE WITH CANNABIS OIL (PAGE 38): ABOUT 25 MG THC PER SERVING

1 (15-ounce) can chickpeas, drained and rinsed

¼ cup plus 2 tablespoons tahini

3 tablespoons freshly squeezed lemon juice (juice of 1 large lemon)

2 tablespoons Cannabis Olive Oil (page 38)

2 tablespoons minced fresh Italian parsley

1 teaspoon minced garlic

¾ teaspoon salt, or to taste

½ teaspoon freshly ground black pepper, or to taste

¼ teaspoon cayenne pepper, or to taste (optional)

1 tablespoon extra-virgin olive oil (optional)

¼ teaspoon paprika (optional)

1. Add the chickpeas, tahini, lemon juice, Cannabis Oil, parsley, garlic, salt, black pepper, and cayenne (if using) to a food processor. Process until smooth. If the hummus is too thick, add a small amount of water, 1 tablespoon at a time, until you reach a consistency you like.

2. Transfer to a serving bowl. Make a small well in the center of the dip and pour in the olive oil (if using) and sprinkle with the paprika (if using). Refrigerate in an airtight container for up to 1 week.

Ingredient Tip Tahini is a butter made from sesame seeds. Find it in health food stores, Middle Eastern markets, and most supermarkets.

GANJA GUACAMOLE
VEGAN, GLUTEN-FREE, DAIRY-FREE, NUT-FREE

SERVES 6

--

PREP TIME:
10 MINUTES

Guacamole is a go-to food for any time of day or night. Serve as a dip with chips or fresh veggies for a snack, or add guacamole to tacos, burritos, quesadillas, or sandwiches. A smooth, cannabis-dosed dollop makes a great accompaniment to grilled chicken, steak, and veggies, too.

DOSAGE WHEN MADE WITH CANNABIS OIL (PAGE 38): ABOUT 25 MG THC PER SERVING

2 medium ripe avocados
1 medium ripe tomato, chopped
¼ cup finely chopped red or yellow onion
1 small scallion, finely chopped
1 medium jalapeño pepper, cored, seeded, and minced
2 tablespoons finely chopped cilantro
1 tablespoon Cannabis Oil (page 38)
1 tablespoon freshly squeezed lime juice
¼ teaspoon minced garlic
Salt
Freshly ground black pepper

1. Peel and pit the avocados and place them in a food processor along with the tomato, onion, scallion, jalapeño, cilantro, Cannabis Oil, lime juice, garlic, salt, and black pepper. Pulse until the ingredients are evenly combined and texture is almost smooth.

2. Season with additional salt and pepper if necessary.

Preparation tip To evenly distribute the cannabis in the avocado, mash this dip a bit more than you might when making an unmedicated, perhaps chunkier, guacamole.

HOT SPINACH DIP
VEGETARIAN, NUT-FREE

SERVES 8

—

PREP TIME:
15 MINUTES

—

BAKE TIME:
30 MINUTES

The unique flavor of spinach blends beautifully with cream cheese in this classic, warm party dip. It's so good and so tempting, no one will raise an eyebrow if you turn it into a full meal, especially when it's served with crusty bread.

DOSAGE WHEN MADE WITH CANNABIS OIL (PAGE 38): ABOUT 20 MG THC PER SERVING

1½ **pounds fresh baby spinach**
1 **to 2 jalapeño peppers**
2 **scallions**
¼ **teaspoon minced garlic**
4 **ounces cream cheese**
¾ **cup grated Parmesan cheese, divided**
¼ **cup mayonnaise**
1 **tablespoon Cannabis Oil (page 38)**
2 **teaspoons soy sauce**
1 **teaspoon freshly squeezed lemon juice**
¼ **teaspoon cayenne pepper (optional)**
Salt
Freshly ground black pepper
Crusty bread or crackers for serving

1. Preheat the oven to 375°F.

2. Wash the spinach. Place the wet spinach in a skillet over medium-high heat. Cook, stirring often, until the spinach has wilted, about 2 minutes. Remove from the heat and drain, squeezing out as much water as possible. Set aside.

3. Combine the jalapeños, scallions, and garlic in a food processor and process until finely chopped. Add the cream cheese, ½ cup of Parmesan cheese, mayonnaise, Cannabis Oil, soy sauce, lemon juice, cayenne (if using), salt, and black pepper and process until almost smooth. Add the drained spinach and process until coarsely chopped. Season to taste with additional salt and pepper.

4. Place the mixture in a small baking dish and sprinkle the remaining ¼ cup of Parmesan cheese on top. Bake about 25 minutes, or until bubbly and the top is beginning to brown. Serve hot with crusty bread or crackers for dipping.

Substitution Tip For hot artichoke dip, swap out the spinach for an 11-ounce can of water-packed artichoke hearts. No need to cook them, just add the drained artichoke hearts to the food processor, blend, and bake.

SWEET AND SPICY MIXED NUTS
VEGETARIAN, GLUTEN-FREE

SERVES 6

—

PREP TIME:
10 MINUTES

—

BAKE TIME:
30 MINUTES

Adjust the amount of cayenne pepper in this recipe up or down depending on your heat tolerance. A nice little spicy bite on the finish is what we're aiming for. The sweetness from the brown sugar makes a great counterbalance to the kick of the cayenne.

DOSAGE WHEN MADE WITH CANNABIS BUTTER (PAGE 37): ABOUT 25 MG THC PER SERVING

2 tablespoons unsalted butter, plus additional (optional) to grease the baking sheet
1 tablespoon Cannabis Butter (page 37)
¼ cup packed dark brown sugar
1 tablespoon water
⅛ to ¼ teaspoon cayenne pepper
3 cups mixed salted nuts

1. Preheat the oven to 300°F. Line a large baking sheet with parchment paper, or alternatively, generously grease with butter.

2. In a small saucepan over medium heat, combine the butter, Cannabis Butter, brown sugar, water, and cayenne. Bring to a boil, stirring constantly, and cook for about 20 seconds.

3. Place the nuts in a medium bowl. Pour in the sauce and toss to combine and evenly coat the nuts.

4. Spread the coated nuts in a single layer on the prepared baking sheet. Bake for 10 minutes. Stir the nuts to break up pieces and return to the oven for 15 more minutes. Let cool slightly before serving. Store for 1 week or longer in an airtight container at room temperature.

Substitution Tip Substitute small pretzels for the nuts in this sweet and spicy snack mix—or combine half nuts and half pretzels for the best of both worlds.

CARAMEL CORN
VEGETARIAN, GLUTEN-FREE, NUT-FREE

SERVES 4

—

PREP TIME:
10 MINUTES

—

BAKE TIME:
15 MINUTES

This is perhaps the most crave-worthy recipe I have ever created. Portion out this salty-sweet concoction carefully, otherwise eating too much is inevitable. It's a great grab-and-go snack when you're in a hurry.

DOSAGE WHEN MADE WITH CANNABIS BUTTER (PAGE 37): ABOUT 20 MG THC PER SERVING

3 quarts (12 cups) plain popped popcorn

⅓ cup unsalted butter, plus additional (optional) for greasing baking sheets

1 tablespoon Cannabis Butter (page 37)

1 cup packed dark brown sugar

¼ cup honey

2 teaspoons salt (preferably sea salt), divided

¾ teaspoon baking soda

1 teaspoon vanilla or maple extract

1. Preheat the oven to 225°F. Line 2 large baking sheets with parchment paper or grease generously with butter.

2. Place the popcorn in a large bowl.

3. In a medium saucepan over medium heat, melt the butter and Cannabis Butter. Stir in the brown sugar, honey, and ½ teaspoon of salt and cook, stirring constantly, until the mixture comes to a boil.

4. Lower the heat to a simmer. If you have a candy thermometer, cook until the mixture reaches 250°F, otherwise you can get close by cooking for about 1½ minutes.

5. Remove the pan from the heat and quickly stir in the baking soda and vanilla, which will turn the mixture into a light brown froth. Working quickly before the caramel cools and starts to harden, pour over the popcorn and toss and stir until evenly coated.

Continued

6. Spread the caramel-coated popcorn in a single layer on the prepared baking sheets and sprinkle on the remaining 1½ teaspoons of salt.

7. Bake for 15 minutes, then stir the popcorn to break up pieces and return to the oven for 15 minutes more. Let cool slightly before serving. For longer storage, cool completely and place in an airtight container for about 1 week.

Preparation tip You can use an air popper, regular popcorn maker, or the stovetop to make the popcorn for this recipe—follow the directions on the popcorn package or that came with your appliance. You can even use store-bought plain popcorn. Avoid microwave popcorn as it has too many other flavors, fats, and salts that will compete with the delicate caramel.

KALE CHIPS
VEGAN, GLUTEN-FREE, DAIRY-FREE, NUT-FREE

Today's hottest health food snack is outrageously expensive to buy, but cheap and simple to make. This recipe is one of the easiest and healthiest ways to use cannabis-infused oil, and these chips are the perfect snack.

DOSAGE WHEN MADE WITH CANNABIS OIL (PAGE 38): ABOUT 25 MG THC PER SERVING

12 ounces fresh kale
2 tablespoons Cannabis Olive Oil (page 38)
1 teaspoon seasoning salt

1. Preheat the oven to 250°F.

2. Wash the kale well to remove any dirt. Keeping the leaves as large as possible, cut or tear the leaves from the tough stems. Dry the leaves well using a clean kitchen towel or paper towels.

3. Place the kale leaves in a large bowl, drizzle with the Cannabis Oil, and toss to coat. Sprinkle with the seasoning salt and toss again.

4. Spread the leaves in a single layer on two large baking sheets, taking care not to overcrowd them. Bake for about 25 minutes, rotating the baking sheets once halfway through baking. The finished leaves will still be intact but completely dry to the touch.

5. Cool completely. Store leftovers in an airtight container for about 1 week.

Variation tip For Italian-style Kale Chips, omit the seasoning salt and sprinkle with 2 teaspoons of freshly ground black pepper and ⅓ cup of grated Parmesan cheese. For Asian-style Kale Chips, substitute cannabis vegetable oil for the olive oil and add 1 teaspoon of toasted sesame oil; omit the seasoning salt and substitute 1 teaspoon of table salt and 2 tablespoons of sesame seeds.

SLICED APPLES WITH CARAMEL DIP

VEGETARIAN, GLUTEN-FREE, NUT-FREE

Here's a tantalizing treat that's reminiscent of the caramel apples we loved as kids—but a lot less messy to eat. The crisp texture and tartness of the apples are a natural pairing for the rich, gooey-sweet caramel. Great apples can be found all year round, but nothing beats their taste in autumn when they're in season.

DOSAGE WHEN MADE WITH CANNABIS BUTTER (PAGE 37): ABOUT 20 MG THC PER SERVING

¾ **cup brown sugar**

¾ **cup sugar**

½ **cup corn syrup**

⅓ **cup unsalted butter**

**1 tablespoon Cannabis Butter
 (page 37)**

½ **teaspoon salt**

⅔ **cup heavy (whipping) cream**

**4 large apples, peeled and sliced
 for dipping**

1. Place the brown and white sugars, corn syrup, butter, Cannabis Butter, and salt in a medium saucepan over medium heat. Cook, stirring occasionally, until the mixture comes to a full boil, about 5 minutes. Lower the heat to a simmer and cook about 2 more minutes.

2. Remove the pan from the heat and stir in the cream until well blended. The caramel will thicken as it cools.

3. Serve as a warm or chilled dip with apple slices. Leftovers will keep in the fridge in an airtight container for several days, if you can resist them that long.

Substitution tip To make this recipe with Cannabis Cream (page 39) instead of butter, use all nonmedicated butter and add 1 tablespoon of Cannabis Cream to the cream that is stirred into the caramel in step 2.

DEVILED EGGS

VEGETARIAN, GLUTEN-FREE, DAIRY-FREE, NUT-FREE

SERVES 6

PREP TIME:
15 MINUTES

COOK TIME:
14 MINUTES

An old-fashioned favorite gets a modern update with a dose of cannabis. These deviled eggs can be more than your average snack. Enjoy them as a satisfying breakfast, packed up for a light lunch, or paired with a salad for dinner.

DOSAGE WHEN MADE WITH 60% THC KIEF: ABOUT 25 MG THC PER SERVING

6 hard-boiled eggs
3 tablespoons mayonnaise
¾ teaspoon Dijon mustard
¾ teaspoon prepared horseradish
¾ teaspoon apple cider vinegar
¼ teaspoon sugar
Salt
Freshly ground black pepper
¼ gram decarboxylated kief
⅛ teaspoon paprika

1. Cut the eggs in half lengthwise and carefully scoop out the yolks into a small bowl.

2. To the bowl, add the mayonnaise, mustard, horseradish, cider vinegar, sugar, salt, pepper, and kief. Use a fork to mix and mash everything together until it is well mixed and mostly smooth.

3. Use a teaspoon to spoon the egg yolk mixture into the egg whites. Sprinkle lightly with the paprika. Refrigerate until ready to serve.

Ingredient Tip For foolproof, perfect, easy-to-peel hard-boiled eggs every time, bring 1 quart of water and 1 tablespoon of distilled white vinegar to a boil. Gently add the eggs and cook for 15 minutes. Place the hot boiled eggs in a large bowl of ice water. Peel as soon as the eggs are cool enough to handle.

ONION DIP

VEGETARIAN, GLUTEN-FREE, NUT-FREE

SERVES 6

—

PREP TIME:
5 MINUTES

—

COOK TIME:
20 MINUTES

Everyone's favorite party dip is even more popular when it teams up with cannabis. Try this one as a tasty match for chips and fresh, raw veggies. Whether you're watching a game or hanging out at a backyard barbecue, this dip will hit the spot.

DOSAGE WHEN MADE WITH MARIJUANA MAYONNAISE (PAGE 44): ABOUT 25 MG THC PER SERVING

2 tablespoons extra-virgin olive oil

1½ cups diced white or yellow onions

1½ cups sour cream

6 tablespoons Marijuana Mayonnaise (page 44)

6 tablespoons mayonnaise

1 teaspoon salt

½ teaspoon garlic powder

½ teaspoon freshly ground black pepper

1. Heat the olive oil in large skillet over medium heat. Add the onions and cook, stirring occasionally, until they are caramelized, about 20 minutes. Remove the pan from the heat and set aside to cool.

2. In a medium bowl, mix the sour cream, Marijuana Mayonnaise, mayonnaise, salt, garlic powder, and pepper together until smooth.

3. Stir the cooled onions into the sour cream mixture. Refrigerate in an airtight container for up to 5 days.

Ingredient Tip While any type of yellow or white onion can be used, for best flavor choose a sweet variety, such as Maui or Vidalia.

POT PARTY CHEX MIX
VEGETARIAN

SERVES 6

—

PREP TIME:
15 MINUTES

—

COOK TIME:
50 MINUTES

Once you start snacking on this cannabis-fortified party mix, it's hard to stop—so keep an eye on your portions to avoid overdoing it. The lively mix of flavors and textures from the cereal, crackers, pretzels, and peanuts make it irresistible. The fact that it's so easy to make is an extra perk.

DOSAGE WHEN MADE WITH CANNABIS BUTTER (PAGE 37): ABOUT 25 MG THC PER SERVING

3 cups Chex cereal, corn, rice, wheat, or a mix

1 cup bite-size Cheddar crackers

1 cup thin pretzel sticks

1 cup roasted peanuts

2 tablespoons Cannabis Butter (page 37)

2 tablespoons unsalted butter

2 tablespoons Worcestershire sauce

1 teaspoon seasoned salt

¾ teaspoon garlic powder

¾ teaspoon onion powder

⅛ teaspoon cayenne pepper (optional)

1. Preheat the oven to 250°F.

2. Combine the cereal, crackers, pretzels, and peanuts in a large bowl. Spread the mix in an even layer on a large baking sheet.

3. Melt the Cannabis Butter and butter in a small saucepan over low heat. Whisk in the Worcestershire sauce, seasoned salt, garlic powder, onion powder, and cayenne (if using).

4. Pour the butter mixture over the cereal mixture and stir to coat the ingredients.

5. Bake for 50 minutes, stirring the mix every 10 to 15 minutes. Let cool completely, then store in an airtight container or portion into sealable plastic bags for up to 2 weeks.

Substitution tip Depending on your dietary requirements or what's in your cupboard, you can use cannabis-infused butter or olive oil for this recipe interchangeably.

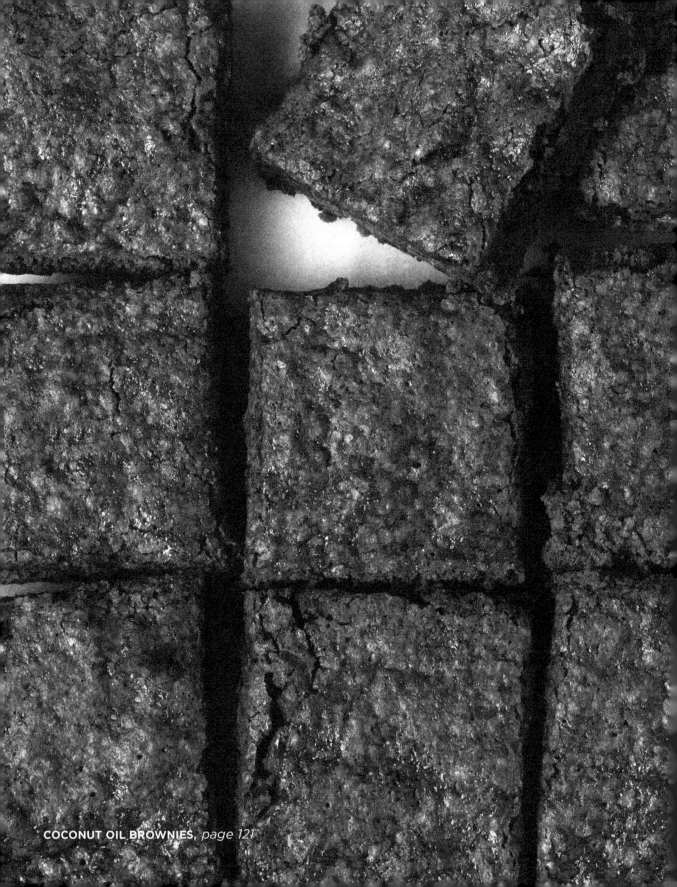

COCONUT OIL BROWNIES, *page 121*

CHAPTER 9
DESSERTS

CLASSIC CHOCOLATE CHIP COOKIES

VEGETARIAN, NUT-FREE

MAKES 30 COOKIES

PREP TIME: 15 MINUTES

BAKE TIME: 10 MINUTES

Since chocolate chip cookies are one of the world's favorites, I thought it was about time to introduce a cannabis-infused version of this classic treat. You can prep and freeze the dough, then bake off smaller batches when the craving hits. For best keeping, portion out the unbaked dough and freeze it between layers of waxed paper in an airtight container.

DOSAGE WHEN MADE WITH CANNABIS BUTTER (PAGE 37): ABOUT 10 MG THC PER COOKIE

⅔ cup sugar

⅔ cup brown sugar

¼ cup Cannabis Butter (page 37), at room temperature

¼ cup unsalted butter, at room temperature

1 teaspoon vanilla extract

1 egg

1⅛ cups all-purpose flour

½ teaspoon baking soda

½ teaspoon salt

1 cup chocolate chips

1. Preheat the oven to 375°F.

2. Beat the sugar, brown sugar, Cannabis Butter, butter, and vanilla extract in a large mixer bowl until creamy. Beat in the egg.

3. Stir together the flour, baking soda, and salt in a small bowl. Gradually beat the dry ingredients into the butter mixture until just incorporated.

4. Stir in the chocolate chips.

5. Drop rounded tablespoons of dough onto 2 ungreased baking sheets, about 1 inch apart. Bake until golden brown, 12 to 15 minutes. Remove and cool on a wire rack immediately.

Substitution Tip These cookies are great with all kinds of add-ins—not just chocolate chips. Mix and match to suit your taste: toasted nuts, white chocolate chips, peanut butter chips, toffee chips, M&M candies, and toasted coconut.

CHOCOLATE PEANUT BUTTER CUP COOKIES

VEGETARIAN

Using a mini-muffin pan allows you to bake up tiny cookie cups filled with rich, dark chocolate ganache. It makes dosing super easy as each person can eat the number of cannabis confections they need.

DOSAGE WHEN MADE WITH CANNABIS BUTTER (PAGE 37): ABOUT 20 MG THC PER COOKIE

Nonstick cooking spray
1 cup sugar
½ cup Cannabis Butter (page 37)
½ cup creamy peanut butter
1 egg
½ teaspoon vanilla extract
1¼ cups all-purpose flour
¾ teaspoon baking soda
½ teaspoon salt
1 cup heavy (whipping) cream
10 ounces dark chocolate chips
   or chunks

1. Preheat the oven to 325°F. Spray 24 mini-muffin tins with the cooking spray.

2. Use an electric mixer to beat together the sugar, Cannabis Butter, and peanut butter until fluffy. Beat in the egg and vanilla extract.

3. In a small bowl, combine the flour, baking soda, and salt, then mix these dry ingredients into the wet ingredients until just combined, forming a dough. Do not overmix.

4. Use clean hands to roll 1 tablespoon each of dough into balls. Place one dough ball in each muffin cup. Form a cup shape by pressing your thumb into each dough ball to make an indentation. The cookies will rise and fill in as they bake; this step makes it easier to mold them later.

5. Bake until lightly browned, about 15 minutes.

Continued

6. Remove the cookies from the oven and use a small spoon to press into the cookie, forming a cup. You *must* do this while the cookies are still hot and pliable. Cool them in the pan for about 10 minutes before removing to a wire rack to cool completely before filling.

7. In a small saucepan, bring the cream to a boil over medium-high heat, watching carefully as it can boil over very quickly. Put the chocolate chips in a small bowl and pour the heated cream over them. Do not stir. Let the mixture sit for about 10 minutes, then whisk until smooth and well combined. Scrape the bottom and sides of the bowl with a rubber spatula to make sure all the chocolate is combined and not stuck to the bottom.

8. Pour the ganache into a pastry bag or small zip-top plastic bag with one small corner snipped off. Pipe the ganache into each cooled cookie cup. Refrigerate in an airtight container for up to 3 days.

Make-ahead Tip These cookies are perfect to prepare in advance and keep in your freezer for anytime you want a medicated treat. Stack them between layers of waxed paper in an airtight, plastic, freezer-safe container. Then remove just the amount you want, bring to room temperature, and enjoy.

CHEESECAKE BROWNIES
VEGETARIAN, NUT-FREE

MAKES 12
BROWNIES
--
PREP TIME:
25 MINUTES
--
BAKE TIME:
30 MINUTES

This medicated brownie combines the best of both words—rich, creamy cheesecake and dark, fudgy brownies melded together in a beautiful, marble swirl. Enjoy with a cold glass of milk or a hot cup of coffee for a satisfying end to any meal.

DOSAGE WHEN MADE WITH CANNABIS BUTTER (PAGE 37): ABOUT 25 MG THC PER SERVING

FOR THE BROWNIE LAYER

Butter, at room temperature, for greasing the pan

¼ cup Cannabis Butter (page 37)

¼ cup plus 2 tablespoons unsalted butter

4 ounces bittersweet or semisweet chocolate

¾ cup granulated sugar

2 large eggs

1 teaspoon vanilla extract

½ cup all-purpose flour

¼ teaspoon salt

FOR THE CHEESECAKE LAYER

8 ounces cream cheese

¼ cup granulated sugar

1 egg

1 tablespoon heavy (whipping) cream or milk

½ teaspoon vanilla extract

TO MAKE THE BROWNIE LAYER

1. Preheat the oven to 350°F. Line an 8-inch-square baking pan with aluminum foil, leaving a couple of inches of over-hang. Grease the foil with butter.

2. Melt the Cannabis Butter, butter, and chocolate over low heat in a medium saucepan, stirring frequently. Set aside to cool for 5 minutes.

3. Stir the sugar into the chocolate until well combined.

4. Beat in the eggs and vanilla extract and continue mixing until well incorporated.

5. Mix in the flour and salt until just incorporated.

6. Reserve ½ cup of the brownie batter and spread the remainder into the prepared pan.

Continued

FOR THE CHEESECAKE LAYER

1. Beat the cream cheese with an electric mixer until smooth. Beat in the sugar, egg, cream, and vanilla extract until smooth and well combined.

2. Spread the cheesecake batter evenly over the brownie batter in the pan.

3. Spoon dollops of the reserved brownie batter over the cheese-cake batter.

4. Use a wooden skewer or the tip of a knife to swirl the dollops of brownie batter into the cheesecake batter. No matter how you do it, it will look decorative.

5. Bake for about 30 minutes, or until a toothpick inserted in the center comes out with just a few moist crumbs cling-ing to it.

6. Let cool in the pan before using the foil to lift out the brownies and slice.

Serving Tip For the best presentation, keep a glass of very hot water next to you when slicing the brownies. Dip the knife in hot water and wipe it off with a paper towel between cuts in order to make neat, clean slices.

COCONUT OIL BROWNIES
VEGETARIAN, DAIRY-FREE

MAKES 12
BROWNIES
—
PREP TIME:
10 MINUTES
—
BAKE TIME:
30 MINUTES

Coconut oil replaces traditional butter in this fudgy brownie recipe, resulting in treats that are both flavorful and super moist. Coconut oil is a surprisingly versatile ingredient for cooking and baking. It doesn't impart all that much coconut flavor to the finished dish, making it a great option for savory recipes, too.

DOSAGE WHEN MADE WITH CANNABIS OIL (PAGE 38): ABOUT 25 MG THC PER SERVING

Vegetable shortening or unsalted butter, at room temperature
¾ cup all-purpose flour
2 tablespoons cocoa powder
¾ teaspoon salt
⅓ cup coconut oil
¼ cup Cannabis Coconut Oil (page 38)
4½ ounces unsweetened chocolate
1 cup packed brown sugar
3 eggs
½ teaspoon vanilla extract
¾ cup chopped macadamia nuts, pecans, or almonds (optional)

1. Preheat the oven to 350°F. Line an 8-inch-square baking pan with aluminum foil, leaving a couple of inches of overhang. Grease the foil with the vegetable shortening.

2. Combine the flour, cocoa powder, and salt in a medium bowl.

3. In a medium saucepan, melt the coconut oil, Cannabis Coconut Oil, and chocolate together over low heat, stirring frequently. Set aside to cool for 5 minutes.

4. Stir the brown sugar into the melted chocolate.

5. Beat in the eggs and vanilla extract and continue mixing until well incorporated.

6. Add in the flour mixture and combine until just incorporated.

7. Stir in nuts (if using).

Continued

8. Pour the batter into the prepared pan and bake for 25 to 30 minutes, or until a toothpick inserted in the center comes out with just a few moist crumbs clinging to it.

9. Let cool in the pan before using the foil to lift out the brownies and slice.

Serving Tip Turn these simple brownies into a spectacular sundae by placing a brownie in a bowl and topping with a scoop of vanilla ice cream. Drizzle with hot fudge sauce and top with whipped cream and a cherry.

RED VELVET CUPCAKES WITH CREAM CHEESE ICING

VEGETARIAN, NUT-FREE

MAKES 24 CUPCAKES
--
PREP TIME: 10 MINUTES
--
BAKE TIME: 20 MINUTES

Because of its dramatic look, red velvet cake always elicits wows from guests, and this cupcake version is no exception. The cocoa powder, buttermilk, and vinegar are what make this cake unique and bring out the natural red color in the cocoa (along with a bit of red coloring).

DOSAGE WHEN MADE WITH CANNABIS OIL (PAGE 38): ABOUT 25 MG THC PER SERVING

FOR THE CUPCAKES

1 cup buttermilk
1 cup vegetable or canola oil
½ cup neutral Cannabis Oil (page 38)
2 eggs
2 tablespoons red food coloring
1 teaspoon distilled white vinegar
1 teaspoon vanilla extract
2½ cups all-purpose flour
1½ cups sugar
6 tablespoons cocoa powder
1 teaspoon baking soda
¾ teaspoon salt

FOR THE ICING

8 ounces cream cheese, at room temperature
½ cup unsalted butter, at room temperature
1 teaspoon vanilla extract
3½ cups confectioners' sugar

TO MAKE THE CUPCAKES

1. Preheat the oven to 350°F. Line 24 muffin cups with paper cupcake liners.

2. In a large bowl, beat together the buttermilk, vegetable oil, Cannabis Oil, eggs, food coloring, vinegar, and vanilla extract with an electric mixer.

3. In a medium bowl, stir together the flour, sugar, cocoa powder, baking soda, and salt. Add these dry ingredients to the wet ingredients and mix just until smooth.

4. Divide the batter among the prepared muffin cups, filling each about two-thirds full. Bake until a toothpick inserted in the center of a cake comes out clean, about 20 minutes. Cool completely before icing.

Continued

TO MAKE THE ICING

1. Beat together the cream cheese, butter, and vanilla extract with an electric mixer until light and fluffy. Lower the mixer speed and slowly beat in the confectioners' sugar until fully incorporated. Increase the mixer speed and beat until the icing is light and fluffy.

2. Spread the icing over the top of each cupcake, leaving a small rim unfrosted to allow the cake to peek through.

Storage tip This recipe makes a lot of cupcakes, so you can always freeze some for later. In resealable freezer bags, stack the iced cupcakes between layers of waxed paper and freeze for up to 6 months. Thaw at room temperature or in the refrigerator.

MAKES 24
CUPCAKES
––
PREP TIME:
25 MINUTES
––
BAKE TIME:
20 MINUTES

DEATH BY CHOCOLATE CUPCAKES

VEGETARIAN, NUT-FREE

Decadent, fudgy cupcakes, studded with chocolate chips, are topped with an even richer chocolate and sour cream ganache frosting and chocolate cookie crumbs. If you gotta go, there's no better way than Death by Chocolate!

DOSAGE WHEN MADE WITH CANNABIS OIL (PAGE 38): ABOUT 25 MG THC PER COOKIE

FOR THE CUPCAKES

- **1 (19.25-ounce) box dark chocolate cake mix**
- **1 (2-ounce) box instant chocolate pudding mix**
- **1 cup sour cream**
- **½ cup Cannabis Vegetable or Canola Oil (page 38)**
- **½ cup brewed espresso or strong coffee**
- **4 eggs**
- **2 cups chocolate chips**

FOR THE GANACHE

- **11 ounces good-quality dark chocolate**
- **1 cup sour cream**
- **6 chocolate sandwich cookies, such as Oreos**

TO MAKE THE CUPCAKES

1. Preheat the oven to 350°F. Line 2 muffin tins with paper cupcake liners.

2. Use an electric mixer on low speed to mix together the dry cake and pudding mixes. Mix in the sour cream, Cannabis Oil, espresso, and eggs. Beat until everything is just combined, but do not overmix. The batter will be thick. Fold in the chocolate chips.

3. Fill each muffin cup slightly more than half full.

4. Bake for about 15 minutes, or until the cupcake tops spring back when gently touched. Remove the cupcakes from the tins and cool completely on a wire rack before icing.

Continued

TO MAKE THE GANACHE

1. Chop the chocolate into small pieces and place in the top of a double boiler or in a stainless steel bowl suspended over simmering water. Stir until just melted and smooth. Remove from the heat and let cool slightly before stirring in the sour cream. Chill for 10 minutes.

2. Use a small spatula to spread a generous of layer of ganache on top of each cupcake, going all the way to the edges. Don't worry about being fancy, it will all get covered.

3. Add the chocolate sandwich cookies to a blender or food processor and process into crumbs, or crush by hand by putting the cookies in a plastic bag and using a rolling pin. Dip each frosted cupcake into the crumbs to coat the top. Serve.

Preparation tip An ice cream scoop makes a quick, easy, and mess-free way of filling the paper-lined cups. Like most cupcake recipes, this one freezes well.

MINI PINEAPPLE UPSIDE-DOWN CAKES

VEGETARIAN, NUT-FREE

Caramel-infused pineapple covers moist, delicate cake for an unforgettable meal finale that looks as great as it tastes. For portion control, I've baked these in individual ramekins that conveniently happen to be the exact size of a single slice of pineapple.

DOSAGE WHEN MADE WITH CANNABIS BUTTER (PAGE 37): ABOUT 20 MG THC PER COOKIE

⅓ cup unsalted butter plus 6 tablespoons, at room temperature, divided, plus additional to grease the ramekins

⅔ cup packed brown sugar

8 canned pineapple slices, drained, juice (about ¼ cup) reserved

8 maraschino cherries

½ cup sugar

2 tablespoons Cannabis Butter (page 37), at room temperature

½ cup buttermilk

1½ teaspoons vanilla extract

2 egg yolks

1½ cups all-purpose flour

2 teaspoons baking powder

1 teaspoon cinnamon

¾ teaspoon salt

2 egg whites

1. Preheat the oven to 350°F. Butter 8 (6-ounce/3½-inch diameter) ramekins and place them on a large baking sheet.

2. With an electric mixer on high speed, cream together ⅓ cup of butter and the brown sugar until evenly combined. Divide the mixture between the ramekins and spread it evenly over the bottoms. Place in the oven until the sugar melts, about 10 minutes.

3. Place a pineapple slice in each ramekin and a maraschino cherry in the center of each pineapple slice. Set aside but keep the oven on.

4. In a large bowl, use the electric mixer on high speed to beat together the sugar, Cannabis Butter, and 6 tablespoons of butter until light and fluffy. Beat in the reserved pineapple juice, buttermilk, vanilla extract, and egg yolks until well combined.

Continued

5. In a small bowl, stir together the flour, baking powder, cinnamon, and salt. With the mixer on low speed, beat the dry ingredients into the wet ingredients until just combined.

6. In a clean bowl and with clean beaters, beat the egg whites until stiff peaks form. Stir one-third of the egg whites into the batter to lighten it. Then use a rubber spatula to gently fold the remaining egg whites into the batter just until combined. Divide the batter among the ramekins, almost filling them.

7. Bake for about 25 minutes, or until a toothpick inserted into the cake comes out clean.

8. Immediately invert the ramekins onto a serving platter or individual serving plates and allow them to sit that way for at least 10 minutes. Carefully lift off the ramekins. If any pineapple slices stick to the bottom of the ramekin, simply use a blunt knife to lift it off and place on top of the cake. Serve warm, at room temperature, or cold.

Preparation Tip No ramekins? No problem. This recipe can also be baked as one large cake in a 9-inch cast-iron skillet or a 9-inch baking pan or cake tin.

INDIVIDUAL PEACH COBBLERS
VEGETARIAN, NUT-FREE

MAKES 12 MINI COBBLERS

--

PREP TIME: 20 MINUTES

--

BAKE TIME: 45 MINUTES

I turned a favorite cobbler into cupcakes with this easy recipe that takes the guesswork out of portion control. Nothing tops a fresh, juicy peach in the heat of the summer. If you're like me and have more peaches on hand than you can eat, these snack-size cakes are a great way to use up the extra fruit.

DOSAGE WHEN MADE WITH CANNABIS BUTTER (PAGE 37): ABOUT 25 MG THC PER SERVING

Vegetable shortening or butter, at room temperature, for greasing the pan

¾ cup diced peaches, fresh, canned, or frozen

3 tablespoons sugar plus 1 cup, divided

½ teaspoon cinnamon

1 cup all-purpose flour

1½ teaspoons baking powder

½ teaspoon nutmeg

¼ teaspoon salt

1 cup milk

¼ cup Cannabis Butter (page 37), melted

¼ cup unsalted butter, melted

1 teaspoon vanilla extract

2 teaspoons coarse natural sugar (optional)

Whipped cream or ice cream, for serving (optional)

1. Preheat the oven to 350°F. Grease a 12-muffin tin with the vegetable shortening.

2. In a small bowl, toss the diced peaches with 3 tablespoons of sugar and the cinnamon. Set aside.

3. In a medium bowl, stir together the flour, baking powder, 1 cup of sugar, nutmeg, and salt. Whisk in the milk, Cannabis Butter, butter, and vanilla extract just until smooth and well combined.

4. Fill each muffin tin about half full.

5. Sprinkle the peaches onto the batter, but do not press them in.

6. Sprinkle the tops of the cakes with the coarse sugar (if using), and bake until golden brown, 40 to 45 minutes. Let cool in the tins for 5 minutes, then remove to a cooling rack. Serve warm or cooled with whipped cream or ice cream (if using).

Substitution tip Substitute diced, peeled apples for the peaches to make mini apple cobblers. Omit the cinnamon and substitute blueberries, blackberries, or raspberries for a berry version.

LEMON BLUEBERRY SCONES
VEGETARIAN, NUT-FREE

MAKES 8 SCONES

—

PREP TIME: 25 MINUTES

BAKE TIME: 20 MINUTES

I have always found traditional scones dry and bland—but not these! I kicked up the flavor and moisture with the addition of fresh blueberries and a zesty citrus glaze. Leftovers also make a tasty breakfast on the go.

DOSAGE WHEN MADE WITH CANNABIS BUTTER (PAGE 37): ABOUT 20 MG THC PER SERVING

FOR THE SCONES

Vegetable shortening, for greasing the pan

2 cups all-purpose flour

1 tablespoon baking powder

3 tablespoons sugar

½ teaspoon salt

3 tablespoons cold unsalted butter

2 tablespoons cold Cannabis Butter (page 37)

1 cup fresh blueberries

1 cup heavy (whipping) cream plus 2 tablespoons, divided

FOR THE GLAZE

¼ cup freshly squeezed lemon juice

1¼ cups confectioners' sugar

1 tablespoon unsalted butter

Zest of 1 lemon

2 tablespoons coarse raw sugar (optional)

TO MAKE THE SCONES

1. Preheat the oven to 400°F. Cover a baking sheet with parchment paper, or alternatively grease it with vegetable shortening.

2. Place the flour, baking powder, sugar, and salt in a food processor and pulse to combine. Add the butter and Cannabis Butter and pulse to combine until the mixture turns into coarse crumbs. The aim is to process the dough as little as possible. Transfer the mixture to a medium bowl. If you don't have a food processor, you can use two forks or a pastry blender to cut the butter into the dry ingredients until the mixture resembles coarse crumbs.

3. Gently fold the blueberries into the batter, taking care not to mash them as this will change the dough's color.

4. Make a well in the center of the dough, pour in 1 cup of cream, and gently fold everything together until just incorporated. The goal remains to work the dough as little as possible to keep the scones tender.

5. Turn the dough out on a lightly floured surface and press it together into a rectangular log about 12 by 3 inches.

6. Cut the log in half, then cut the pieces in half again, giving you 4 squares. Cut each square in half on a diagonal to create a triangle shape. Place the triangles on the prepared baking sheet and brush the tops with the remaining 2 tablespoons of cream.

7. Place in the oven and immediately reduce the heat to 375°F. Bake for about 20 minutes, or until lightly browned. Remove to a wire rack to cool.

TO MAKE THE GLAZE

1. While the scones are baking, mix the lemon juice with the confectioners' sugar in a small saucepan over medium-low heat. Heat, stirring constantly, until the sugar has dissolved. Whisk in the butter and lemon zest, and continue whisking until the butter is melted.

2. Place the wire rack with the cooling scones on top of a baking sheet. Spoon the glaze over the tops of the scones, allowing it to soak in as much as possible. Sprinkle with the coarse raw sugar (if using). Serve warm or cooled.

Ingredient Tip Zest is the outermost, brightly colored part of a citrus fruit. Since this is where the essential oils are located, it is also extremely flavorful. To make zest, take a fine grater or Microplane and grate off just the thin outermost peel, avoiding any of the bitter, white inner pith.

INDIVIDUAL LEMON BERRY TRIFLES

VEGETARIAN, NUT-FREE

MAKES 10 TRIFLES

PREP TIME: 25 MINUTES PLUS 30 MINUTES TO COOL

BAKE TIME: 20 MINUTES

Not only are these a delicious dessert to keep or share, but they are perfect to make ahead of time and then easily store or transport since each one comes in its own half-pint mason jar. Leftovers will keep in their covered jars for 3 or 4 days in the fridge.

DOSAGE WHEN MADE WITH CANNABIS BUTTER (PAGE 37): ABOUT 35 MG THC PER SERVING

FOR THE CAKE

Vegetable shortening, for greasing the pan

1¼ cups all-purpose flour, plus additional for dusting the pan

1 teaspoon baking powder

¼ teaspoon baking soda

⅛ teaspoon salt

¼ cup Cannabis Butter (page 37), at room temperature

2 tablespoons unsalted butter, at room temperature

¾ cup sugar

2 eggs

½ cup plain yogurt

2 tablespoons freshly squeezed lemon juice

½ teaspoon lemon extract

½ teaspoon grated lemon zest

FOR THE FILLING

2 cups heavy (whipping) cream

½ cup confectioners' sugar

1 teaspoon lemon extract

½ teaspoon grated lemon zest

2 cups fresh blueberries

2 cups fresh raspberries

TO MAKE THE CAKE

1. Preheat the oven to 350°F. Grease and flour a 9-by-13-inch baking sheet with vegetable shortening.

2. In a small bowl, mix together the flour, baking powder, baking soda, and salt.

3. In large bowl, use an electric mixer at high speed to cream the Cannabis Butter, butter, and sugar together until light and fluffy. Beat in the eggs, one at a time, then the yogurt, lemon juice, lemon extract, and lemon zest.

4. Lower the mixer speed and mix in the dry ingredients until just combined. Use a rubber spatula to scrape the bowl edges and mix by hand to ensure the batter is evenly mixed. Pour the batter into the prepared baking pan and use a spatula to smooth it into one even layer. Bake for about 10 minutes or until lightly browned. Set aside to cool for 30 minutes.

TO MAKE THE FILLING

1. Prepare the lemon cream by whipping together the heavy cream, confectioners' sugar, and lemon extract until stiff peaks start to form. Whip in the lemon zest.

2. Use an upside-down half-pint jar as a cookie cutter and cut 20 circles from the baked cake. Don't worry if you need to piece some of these circles together—once they are layered in the jar, nobody will ever know the difference. This dessert is *very* forgiving.

3. Press one cake circle into the bottom of each of 10 half-pint jars. Add a layer of the berries, followed by a layer of cream, then another cake circle, more berries, and more cream. Garnish with a few fresh berries on top and serve. If making in advance, cover each jar with its lid and refrigerate for up to 4 days.

Variation tip Make chocolate raspberry trifles by using the batter from the Death by Chocolate Cupcakes (page 125) to make the cake. Eliminate the lemon extract and zest from the cream, and sandwich the chocolate cake circles between layers of sweetened whipped cream and fresh raspberries.

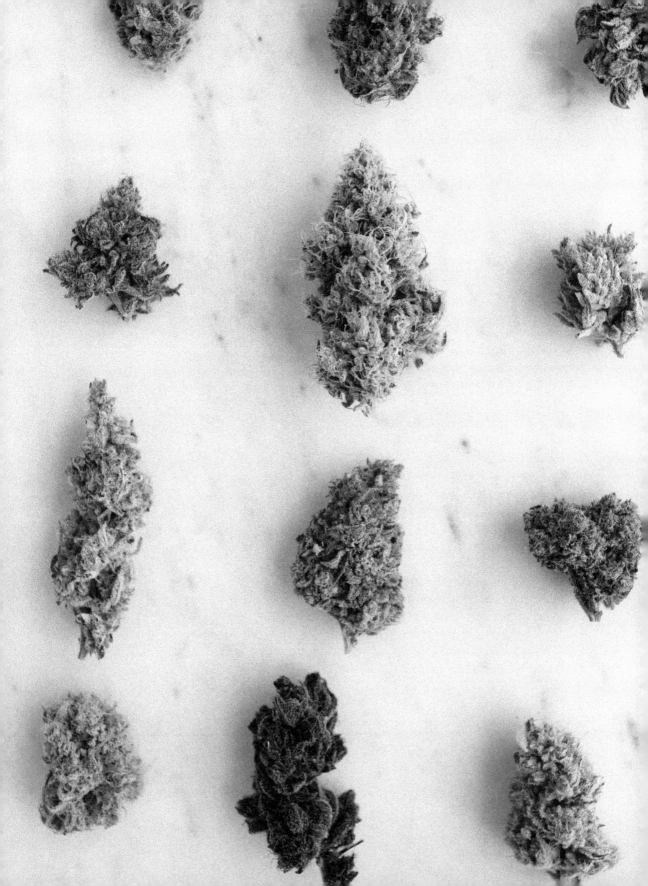

MEASUREMENTS

VOLUME EQUIVALENTS (LIQUID)

US STANDARD	US STANDARD (OUNCES)	METRIC (APPROXIMATE)
2 tablespoons	1 fl. oz.	30 mL
¼ cup	2 fl. oz.	60 mL
½ cup	4 fl. oz.	120 mL
1 cup	8 fl. oz.	240 mL
1½ cups	12 fl. oz	355 mL
2 cups or 1 pint	16 fl. oz.	475 mL
4 cups or 1 quart	32 fl. oz.	1 L
1 gallon	128 fl. oz.	4 L

OVEN TEMPERATURES

FAHRENHEIT (F)	CELSIUS (C) (APPROXIMATE)
250°F	120°C
300°F	150°C
325°F	165°C
350°F	180°C
375°F	190°C
400°F	200°C
425°F	220°C
450°F	230°C

VOLUME EQUIVALENTS (DRY)

US STANDARD	METRIC (APPROXIMATE)
1/8 teaspoon	0.5 mL
¼ teaspoon	1 mL
½ teaspoon	2 mL
¾ teaspoon	4 mL
1 teaspoon	5 mL
1 tablespoon	15 mL
¼ cup	59 mL
1/3 cup	79 mL
½ cup	118 mL
2/3 cup	156 mL
¾ cup	177 mL
1 cup	235 mL
2 cups or 1 pint	475 mL
3 cups	700 mL
4 cups or 1 quart	1 L

WEIGHT EQUIVALENTS

US STANDARD	METRIC (APPROXIMATE)
½ ounce	15 g
1 ounce	30 g
2 ounces	60 g
4 ounces	115 g
8 ounces	225 g
12 ounces	340 g
16 ounces or 1 pound	455 g

GLOSSARY

cannabidiol (CBD): An important nonpsychoactive cannabinoid. CBD can have powerful medicinal effects, and can counter the uncomfortable feeling that may arise after consuming too much THC.

cannabinoids: The natural chemical compounds in cannabis responsible for its medicinal and psychoactive effects. These include THC and CBD, as well as many lesser-known cannabinoids that scientific research is just starting to explore.

decarboxylation: The process of adding heat in order to transform the acidic forms of cannabinoids into their nonacidic forms. Decarboxylation is necessary to convert the nonpsychoactive THCa present in the raw cannabis plant into psychoactive THC.

dispensary: A legal store that sells cannabis and cannabis products.

endocannabinoids: The naturally occurring cannabinoids in the body that all mammals are born with.

endocannabinoid system (ECS): The intricate system of endocannabinoids and cannabinoid receptors in all mammals that help regulate the body's other systems and maintain homeostasis.

fan leaves: Large, pretty leaves of the cannabis plant. While featured in the popular graphic image of marijuana, these leaves are not typically used for smoking or cooking.

flowers: Blooms of the cannabis plant, also known as buds or nugs. This is the prized part of the plant which contains the highest concentration of trichomes.

hash: This concentrate is made by extracting kief (usually with water and ice) from the cannabis plant, then heating and pressing it. Hash consistency can range from light and powdery to sticky and putty-like. It is useful for both smoking and cooking.

hash oil: The collective name for cannabis concentrates extracted with a solvent, usually butane or CO_2. Depending on how it was made, hash oils go by many different names, including shatter, wax, earwax, and budder.

hemp: Cannabis's nonpsychoactive cousin, hemp has been used since the dawn of time in food and as a fiber.

hybrid: A variety of cannabis plant bred by crossing *Cannabis indica* and *Cannabis sativa* in varying ratios. Most marijuana strains found today are in fact hybrids.

indica: A classification of cannabis characterized by short, bushy plants. General wisdom used to say that indica plants delivered more of marijuana's sleepy and relaxing effects, but we are now learning this has more to do with the plant's cannabinoid and terpene profiles.

infusions and extractions: Substances made by extracting cannabinoids from marijuana and infusing them into butter, oil, alcohol, honey, or other substances.

kief: A powder-like substance, containing little to no plant material, made from the resinous trichomes covering the cannabis plant.

sativa: A classification of cannabis characterized by tall plants with thin leaves. General wisdom used to say that sativa plants delivered more of marijuana's energetic and creativity-inducing effects, but we are now learning this has more to do with the plant's cannabinoid and terpene profiles.

shake: The small pieces and bits of marijuana that filter to the bottom of a large bag. When you can find it, shake makes excellent, economical cooking material.

sugar leaves: Tiny, trichome-laden leaves that surround the cannabis flower.

terpenes, terpenoids: The chemical compounds in plants that provide their aroma and are largely responsible for the variety of effects you feel from different marijuana strains.

tetrahydrocannabinol (THC): The cannabinoid in marijuana that produces its psychoactive effects along with a multitude of medicinal effects.

tincture: A concentrated cannabis infusion usually made with alcohol, or occasionally with glycerin.

trichomes: Invisible to the naked eye, these are resinous glands containing cannabinoids and terpenes that cover the marijuana plant. When making a concentrate or an infusion, trichomes are what is extracted.

trim, trimmings: Parts of the cannabis plant that growers remove before selling marijuana. Trimmings consist of fan leaves, sugar leaves, and tiny "popcorn buds" that grow at the base of the plant.

vape, vaporizing: The process of turning plant matter or concentrates into an inhalable vapor, a healthier ingestion method than smoking.

RESOURCES

BOOKS

Armentano, Paul, Steve Fox, and Mason Tvert. *Marijuana Is Safer: So Why Are We Driving People to Drink?* White River Junction, VT: Chelsea Green Publishing, 2013.

Backes, Michael. *Cannabis Pharmacy*. New York: Black Dog & Leventhal Publishers, 2014.

Bienenstock, David. *How to Smoke Pot (Properly): A Highbrow Guide to Getting High.* New York: Plume Publishing, 2016.

Blesching, Uwe. *The Cannabis Health Index: Combining the Science of Medical Marijuana with Mindfulness Techniques to Heal 100 Chronic Symptoms and Diseases.* Berkeley, CA: North Atlantic Books, 2015.

Bobrow, Warren. *Cannabis Cocktails, Mocktails & Tonics: The Art of Spirited Drinks and Buzz-Worthy Libations.* Beverly, MA: Fair Winds Press, 2016.

Cervantes, Jorge. *Marijuana Horticulture: The Indoor/Outdoor Medical Grower's Bible.* Vancouver, WA: Van Patten Publishing, 2006.

Oner, S. T. *Cannabis Indica: The Essential Guide to the World's Finest Marijuana Strains.* San Francisco: Green Candy Press, 2011.

Oner, S. T. *Cannabis Sativa: The Essential Guide to the World's Finest Marijuana Strains.* San Francisco: Green Candy Press, 2012.

Sicard, Cheri. *Mary Jane: The Complete Marijuana Handbook for Women.* Berkeley, CA: Seal Press, 2015.

Werner, Clint. *Marijuana Gateway to Health: How Cannabis Protects Us from Cancer and Alzheimer's Disease.* San Francisco: Dachstar Press, 2011.

Wolf, Laurie. *The Medical Marijuana Dispensary: Understanding, Medicating, and Cooking with Cannabis.* Berkeley, CA: Althea Press, 2016.

WORTHWHILE ORGANIZATIONS

Americans for Safe Access: Safeaccessnow.org

Drug Policy Alliance: Drugpolicy.org

NORML (National Organization for the Reform of Marijuana Laws): NORML.org

Students for Sensible Drug Policy: Ssdp.org

USEFUL WEBSITES

Leafly: General marijuana and dispensary guide site, especially useful for its extensive collection of strain reviews. Leafly.com

Project CBD: An excellent, credible guide to CBD therapy and more. ProjectCBD.org

Recent Research on Medical Applications of Cannabis: NORML does a great job at keeping up with the latest medical research. NORML.org/component/zoo/category /recent-research-on-medical-marijuana

Weedmaps: The largest marijuana dispensary directory. Weedmaps.com

TOOLS & SUPPLIES

Dosage Calculator Tool: Cheri Sicard's online dosing mini-course and homemade edibles dosage calculator tool. bit.ly/dosingcalculator

Making Dry Ice Kief: Two-minute video showing how easy it is to make kief for cooking. www.cannabischeri.com/food/cooking-basics/how-to-make-dry-ice-kief

Kief and Hashmaking: Boldt bags make quality filter bags that will last for years of kief and water hash making. Boldtbags.com

NOVA Decarboxylator: While not essential, this gadget makes perfect decarbing easy and foolproof. Ardentcannabis.com

Magical Butter Machine: Again, not essential, but this gadget makes infusion creation quick, easy, and mess free. The only downside, in my opinion, is it finely grinds the plant material as part of its function. Magicalbutter.com

REFERENCES

Abel, E. L. *Marihuana: The First Twelve Thousand Years.* New York: Plenum Press, 1980.

Armentano, Paul. NORML.org. "Emerging Clinical Applications for Cannabis and Cannabinoids: A Review of the Recent Scientific Literature, Seventh Edition." NORML.org. January 16, 2016. norml.org/pdf_files/NORML_Clinical_Applications_for_Cannabis_and_Cannabinoids.pdf.

Backes, Michael. *Cannabis Pharmacy.* New York: Black Dog & Leventhal Publishers, 2014.

Courtney, William, MD, and Kristen Courtney. "Dietary Benefits of Juicing Raw Cannabis." Lecture, 2011.

El Sohly, Mahmoud A., PhD. "National Institute on Drug Abuse (NIDA) Marijuana Project at the National Center for Natural Products Research." Annual Reports. School of Pharmacy, University of Mississippi. pharmacy.olemiss.edu/marijuana/

Elzinga S., J. Fischedick, R. Podkolinski R, and J. C. Raber. "Cannabinoids and Terpenes as Chemotaxonomic Markers in Cannabis." *Natural Products Chemistry & Research* 3, no. 181 (July 2015). doi:10.4172/2329-6836.1000181.

McDonough, Elise. "Vitamin THC: Cannabis as a Superfood." *High Times.* January 3, 2017. hightimes.com/edibles/vitamin-thc-cannabis-as-a-superfood/

Melamede, Robert, PhD. "Harm Reduction: The Cannabis Paradox." *Harm Reduction Journal* 2, no. 17 (2005). doi:10.1186/1477-7517-2-17.

National Commission on Marihuana and Drug Abuse (NIDA). "Marihuana: A Signal of Misunderstanding, first report." March 1972.

Vandrey, Ryan G., Jeffrey C. Raber, Mark E. Raber, and Marcel Bonn-Miller. "Cannabinoid Dose and Label Accuracy in Edible Marijuana Products." *JAMA* 313, no. 24 (2015): 2491–2493. doi:10.1001/jama.2015.6613.

Werner, Clint. *Marijuana Gateway to Health: How Cannabis Protects Us from Cancer and Alzheimer's Disease.* San Francisco: Dachstar Press, 2011.

RECIPE INDEX

INDEX

ACKNOWLEDGMENTS

No book is possible without the hard work and input of an entire team, and this one is no exception. I sincerely want to thank my amazing editor, Kim Suarez, who did a great job organizing and polishing this book. Thanks as well to Elizabeth Castoria, who brought me this wonderful project, and the entire team at Callisto Media, whose production skills make me look good. I also need to thank everyone who helped me in the writing of this book and put up with me while I wrote it (whether they know it or not), including Tamara Anderson, Paul Armentano, Steve Bloom, Yamileth Bolanos, Chuck and Bambi Burnes, Madison Burnes, Richard and Tracy Burnes, Catrina Coleman, Mara Felsen, Kandice Hawes, Cynthia Johnston, Charles Lynch, Elise McDonough, Dr. Robert Melamede, Mitch Mandell, Clifford Perry, Dr. Jeffrey Raber, Wanda Smith, Susan Soares, Lanny Swerdlow, Norma White, Ian Wright, and as always, Zazou. Special thanks also go to all the students of my countless cannabis cooking classes and lectures, both in person and online. Your questions and feedback over the years gave me the best possible barometer of what information the public needs to know about cannabis cooking.

ABOUT THE AUTHOR

CHERI SICARD was a professional food writer, recipe developer, and cooking instructor long before cannabis entered her life, so it was only natural she started cooking with marijuana after her doctor recommended it for a chronic condition. Soon medical marijuana dispensaries and cannabis organizations were calling on her to teach their patients how to cook with marijuana. The classes proved so popular that Cheri has since launched an online version in order to bring cannabis cooking to a larger audience.

After reviewing her book *Mary Jane: The Complete Marijuana Handbook for Women* (2015, Seal Press), *The Daily Beast* dubbed Cheri the "Martha Stewart of Weed." Cheri writes *Freedom Leaf* magazine's monthly Medicated Munchies column, and her articles and cannabis recipes can also be found in *High Times*, *Herb*, *Civilized*, *Cannabis Now*, and more. Her blog is CannabisCheri.com.

CPSIA information can be obtained
at www.ICGtesting.com
Printed in the USA
LVHW01s1143270318
571165LV00003B/3/P